Want t

Ch

7+ Hours of Video Lectures
15+ Hours of Audio Lectures
TONS of cheat sheets and handouts

Everything you need to know to become a MedMaster

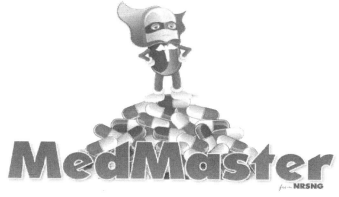

35% OFF Lifetime Membership
Use Coupon Code: 140MEDS

Watch a preview here: https://youtu.be/PBN--MGcJoo

Disclaimer

Medicine and nursing are continuously changing practices. The author and publisher have reviewed all information in this book with resources believed to be reliable and accurate and have made every effort to provide information that is up to date with best practices at the time of publication. Despite our best efforts we cannot disregard the possibility of human error and continual changes in best practices the author, publisher, and any other party involved in the production of this work can warrant that the information contained herein is complete or fully accurate. The author, publisher, and all other parties involved in this work disclaim all responsibility from any errors contained within this work and from the results from the use of this information. Readers are encouraged to check all information in this book with institutional guidelines, other sources, and up to date information. For up to date disclaimer information please visit: http://www.nrsng.com/about.

NCLEX®, NCLEX®-RN ®are registered trademarks of the National Council of State Boards of Nursing, INC. and hold no affiliation or support of this product.

Photo Credits:

All photos are original photos taken or created by the author or rights purchased at Fotolia.com. All rights to appear in this book have been secured.

Some images within this book are either royalty-free images, used under license from their respective copyright holders, or images that are in the public domain. Images used under a creative commons license are duly attributed, and include a link to the relevant license, as per the author's instructions. All Creative Commons images used under the following license. All works in the public domain are considered public domain given life of the author plus 70 years or more as required by United States law.

NCLEX® Essentials - Med Surg
Everything You Need to Know for the NCLEX®

NRSNG.com | NursingStudentBooks.com

Jon Haws RN CCRN
Tarang Patel RN CCRN SRNA
Sandra Haws RD CNSC MS

©**TazKai LLC** NRSNG.com First Edition July 2015

Your Free Gift!

As a way of saying thanks for your purchase, I'm offering a free PDF download:

"63 Must Know NCLEX® Labs"

With these charts you will be able to take the 63 most important labs with you anywhere you go!

You can download the 4 page PDF document by going to NRSNG.com/labs

Contents

Introduction

While every NCLEX® exam is different by nature of computer adaptive testing, this book contains the most important information that will not only aid you in taking the exam, but also in your work as a nurse.

The purpose of this book is to condense the information you need to know into an easy to study and digest format. This is not a complete guide to Med-Surg (that is what text books are for) but rather an attempt to extract only the most vital information.

You should consult this book to review and highlight information as you work your way through nursing school and as you prepare for the NCLEX®.

Many students state that nursing school is "like drinking from a fire hose" . . . I would have to agree with that sentiment. I remember my time in nursing school, not only are you learning how to care for patients but you are learning new skills, a tremendous amount of new information, and essentially a new language . . . it's tough to say the least.

Our goal at NRSNG.com is to simplify your journey. You will still need to put in a huge amount of work, but we think that nursing school can be easier as you learn what exactly you should focus on and forget the fluff.

Enjoy the book. . .

Happy Nursing!

-**Jon Haws** RN BSN CCRN
CEO NRSNG.com

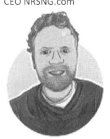

Cardiovascular Disorders

Cardiac Dysrhythmias

	Route			Rate	Rhythm	
Rhythm	P Wave	PR Interval	QRS	Rate	Regularity	Causes
Normal Sinus	Normal	0.12-0.20	<0.12	60-100	Regular	Normal Finding
Sinus Bradycardia	Normal	0.12-0.20	<0.12	<60	Regular	Sleep, inactivity, athletic, vagal tone, drugs, MI, K+, respiratory arrest
Sinus Tachycardia	Normal	0.12-0.20	<0.12	>100, usually 100-150	Regular	Caffeine, exercise, fever, anxiety, heart failure, drugs, pain, hypoxia, hypotension, volume depletion
Atrial Pause	Looks like SR but drops a complex			Normal or slow	Irregular	Elderly, digoxin toxicity, MI,

						rheumatic fever
Atrial Flutter	Saw tooth	None	<0.12	Atrial rate 250-400	Regular or Irregular	Valvular heart disease, MI, CHF, pericarditis
Atrial Fibrillation	Wavy unidentifiable	None	<0.12	Atrial rate >400	Irregular	Heart disease, pulmonary disease, emotional stress, excessive alcohol or caffeine
Junctional Rhythm	INVERTED before or after QRS or absent	<0.12	<0.12	40-60	Regular	Electrical impulse not arriving from SA node, AV node fires at inherent rate
Accelerated Junctional Rhythm	INVERTED before or after QRS or absent	<0.12	<0.12	60-100	Regular	Digoxin toxicity, damage to AV node
Junctional Tachycardia	INVERTED before or after QRS or absent	<0.12	<0.12	>100	Regular	Same as SVT

Supraventricular Tachycardia	Pointed or hidden in T	Immeasurable	<0.12	150-250	Regular	Caffeine, CHF, fatigue, hypoxia, mitral valve disease, altered pacemaker in heart
Idioventricular Rhythm	None	None	>0.11 wide and bizarre	20-40	Regular	Digoxin toxicity, acute MI
Ventricular Tachycardia	None	None	>0.11 wide and bizarre	150-250	Regular	MI, ischemia, digoxin toxicity, hypoxia, acidosis, ↓K+, ↓BP
Ventricular Fibrillation	None	None	None	None	Irregular, vary in size, shape and height	Follow PVC, VT, most common cause of sudden death
Asystole	Possible	None	None	None	No QRS	Follows VT/VFib, acidosis, hypoxia, ↓K+, hypothermia, drug overdose
1° AV Block	Normal	>0.20	<0.12	Varies	Regular or	First sign of

						irregular	increasing AV block
2° AV Block Type I	Normal	Varies: progressively prolonged	<0.12	Varies	Regularly irregular: QRS dropped after progressively prolonged PRI	Acute inferior MI, digoxin toxicity, vagal stimulation, conduction system disease
2° AV Block Type II	Normal	Consistent normal or prolonged	Normal or wide	Usually slow	Regular or irregular; occasionally dropped QRS	BBB, anterior MI, lesions of conduction system
3° AV Block	Normal	No relationship between PR & QRS	Wide	Slow	Regular	Atria and ventricles beat independently, digoxin or K+ toxicity, acute MI, ischemic heart disease
Premature Atrial Contractions	Yes, PAC P wave shaped different	May differ from underlying rhythm	<0.12	Rate of underlying rhythm	PAC complexes come early	Coffee, tea, alcohol, CHF, emotions, fatigue, fever, hypoxia,

						mitral valve disease
Premature Junctional Contractions	Inverted before or after QRS or absent	<0.12	<0.12	Rate of underlying rhythm	PJC make it irregular	Vagal tone, stress, caffeine, alcohol, heart failure, digoxin toxicity, ↓K+
Premature Ventricular Contractions	None	N/A	>0.11 wide and bizarre	Dependant on underlying rhythm	Irregular due to premature beat	Ventricular irritability, hypoxia, ↓K+, Ca, MI, digoxin toxicity, anxiety

Sinus Bradycardia

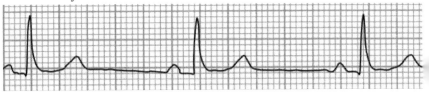

Sinus bradycardia is essentially the result of the SA node initiating impulses at a slower rate than normal. Conduction follows the correct path but at a slower rate.

1. Overview
    a. Rhythm is regular
    b. Rate <60
2. NCLEX® Points
    a. Therapeutic Management

     i.   Determine cause

     ii.   Atropine may be administered to keep the rate >60

     iii.   Monitor hemodynamics, insure proper CO

     iv.   permanent pacemaker may be required

Premature Ventricular Contractions (PVC's)

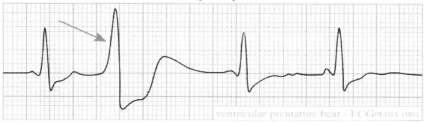

1.   Overview
   a.   early ventricular beats due to irritable ventricles
   b.   may occur in repetitive pattern (bigeminy, trigemeny, quadrigeminy)
2.   NCLEX® Points
   a.   Therapeutic Management
      i.   determine cause
      ii.   assess for hypoxia
      iii.   assess potassium level
      iv.   notify physician if client complains of pain, increased frequency, R on T, multifocal

Ventricular Tachycardia

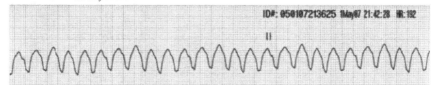

1.   Overview
   a.   irritable ventricles leas to repetitive firing of the ventricles
   b.   may lead to cardiac arrest
2.   NCLEX® Points

a. **ASSESS for pulse first**
  i. Pulse
    1. Administer O2
    2. Administer antidysrhythimcs
    3. notify physician
    4. cardioversion may be required
  ii. No Pulse
    1. Begin ACLS protocol

Ventricular Fibrillation

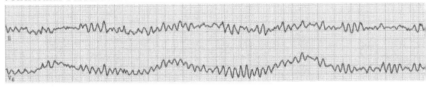

1. Overview
   a. ventricles quiver due to multiple irritable foci
   b. no cardiac output
   c. lethal rhythm
2. NCLEX® Points
   a. Therapeutic Interventions
     i. Begin ACLS protocol immediately
     ii. assess pulse and rhythm after 2 minutes of compressions

Myocardial Infarction

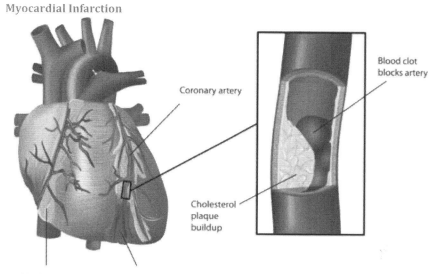

Coronary artery

Blood clot blocks artery

Cholesterol plaque buildup

Healthy heart muscle   Dead heart muscle

1. Overview
    a. Sudden restriction of blood supply to a portion of the heart.
2. NCLEX® Points
    a. Modifiable risk factors
        i. smoking
        ii. obesity
        iii. stress
        iv. ↑Chol
        v. Diabetes
        vi. HTN
    b. Angina Pectoris: chest pain due to restricted blood flow
        i. Stable angina: predictable with increased activity
        ii. Unstable angina: at rest and with activity
        iii. Prinzmetal angina: caused by vasospasm
    c. Nursing Assessment
        i. Chest pain unrelieved by rest
        ii. Crushing chest pain, diaphoresis, mottled skin, nausea, anxiety, SOB, palpitations
        iii. ST elevation on 12-lead

              iv.   Elevated Troponins (most sensitive), elevated CK-MB

      d.   Treatment

           i.   MONA

                1.   morphine, oxygen, nitroglycerin, aspirin

                      a.   Morphine - relieve chest pain

                      b.   Oxygen - increase oxygenation

                      c.   Nitrates - dilate coronary vessels - increase blood supply

                      d.   Aspirin - antiplatelet

           ii.   Monitor EKG

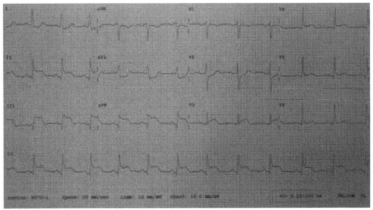

ST Elevation MI

          iii.   Rest - decrease O2 demands of heart

Heart Failure

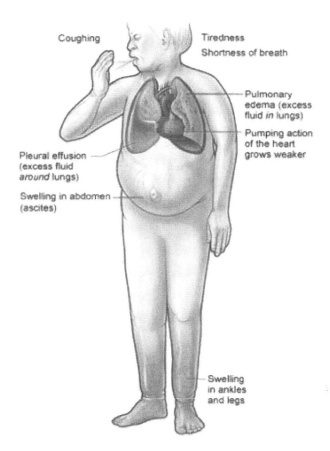

Coughing

Tiredness
Shortness of breath

Pulmonary
edema (excess
fluid *in* lungs)

Pumping action
of the heart
grows weaker

Pleural effusion
(excess fluid
around lungs)

Swelling in abdomen
(ascites)

Swelling
in ankles
and legs

1. Overview
   a. Heart is unable to pump enough blood to the body. Any condition that affects the hearts ability to pump can lead to Heart Failure (MI, valve disorders, HTN, pulmonary HTN).
   b. Initially presents as Right or Left side as it progresses both sides are affected.
   c. **Left Side**
      i. Left ventricle is unable to pump blood into the systemic circulation causing a "back-up" into the pulmonary circulation.

      d. **Right Side**

        i. Right ventricle is unable to pump blood into the pulmonary circulation causing a "back-up" in venous circulation.

2. NCLEX® Points

    a. Nursing Care

      i. raise head of bed

      ii. administer O2

      iii. Assess lung sounds

      iv. Encourage rest

      v. Monitor daily weights

      vi. Instruct on low sodium diet

    b. Medical Management

      i. Diuretics

      ii. Digoxin - improve contractility (CO) (assess apical pulse for 1 full minute)

      iii. ACE Inhibitors - decrease afterload (increase CO)

Right-Sided Failure	Left-Sided Failure
Systemic circulation	Pulmonary circulation
Dependent edema	Dyspnea
JVD	Crackles in lungs
Abdominal distention	Tachypnea

Valve Disorders

1. Overview

    a. Valves do not open (stenosis) or close (regurgitation) completely

    b. blood flow is jeopardized

2. NCELX® Points

    a. Types

      i. Mitral Stenosis

        1. mitral valve does not open completely during diastole

      ii. Mitral regurgitation

        1. Mitral valve does not close completely before systole

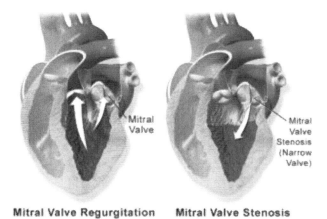

Mitral Valve Regurgitation   Mitral Valve Stenosis

   iii. Aortic Stenosis
      1. aortic valve does not open completely during systole
   iv. Aortic Regurgitation
      1. aortic valve does not close completely prior to diastole

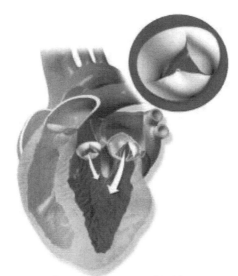

Aortic Regurgitation

Blausen.com staff. "Blausen gallery 2014". Wikiversity Journal of Medicine. DOI:10.15347/wjm/2014.010. ISSN 20018762. (Own work) [CC BY 3.0 (http://creativecommons.org/licenses/by/3.0)], via Wikimedia Commons

- b. Therapeutic Management
    - i. Balloon valvuloplasty
    - ii. Valve replacement
        1. Mechanical: lifetime anticoagulant therapy indicated
        2. Biological: valve from other species
        3. post op
            - a. monitor hemodynamics
            - b. monitor for signs of bleeding
            - c. maintain good oral hygiene with soft bristle tooth brush
            - d. prophylactic antibiotics required prior to invasive procedures
            - e. instruct client on anticoagulant therapy
            - f. avoid dental procedures for 6 months

Endocarditis

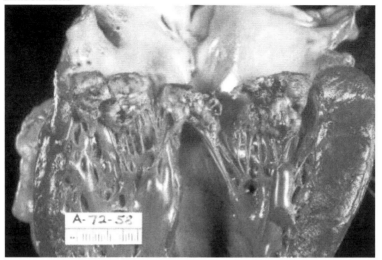

Mitral valve vegetation caused by bacterial endocarditis

1. Overview
    a. inflammation of the inner lining of the heart and valves
    b. common causes include IV drug use and valve replacement
    c. **Vegetations** form which are masses of platelets, fibrin, microorganisms, and inflammatory cells
        i. vegetations can become embolic
    d. infecting organism enters via:
        i. oral cavity (higher risk with recent dental procedure)
        ii. invasive procedures
        iii. infections
2. NCLEX® Points
    a. Assessment
        i. spiking fever
        ii. signs of heart failure
        iii. elevated WBC
        iv. heart murmurs
        v. Embolic complications from vegetations
            1. Splinter hemorrhages in nail beds
            2. Janeway lesions on fingers, toes, nose
            3. Clubbing of fingers

b. Therapeutic Management
  i. Antiembolic stockings
  ii. IV antibiotic therapy
  iii. Oral hygiene with soft bristled tooth brush twice a day and rinse
  iv. Teach client to monitor for signs of infection
  v. Monitor for signs of emboli
  vi. Instruct dental provider of condition (prophylactic antibiotics needed)

Pericarditis

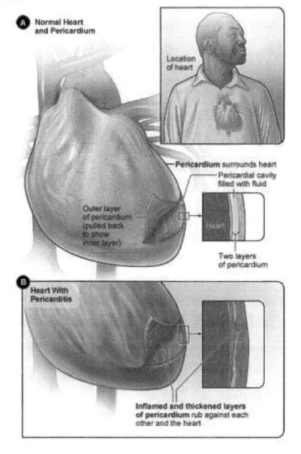

1. Overview

        a.   inflammation of the pericardium

        b.   compression of the heart occurs as the pericardial sac inflames

        c.   heart failure or cardiac tamponade can occur

2. NCLEX® Points

    a.   Assessment

        i.   Pain

            1.   chest radiating to left side of neck, shoulder, or back

            2.   aggravated by inspiration, coughing, and swallowing

            3.   worse in supine position, relieved by leaning forward

        ii.   ST elevation

        iii.   Signs of heart failure

    b.   Therapeutic Management

        i.   assess and treat pain

        ii.   administer O2 and place client in high Fowler's

        iii.   Assess for cardiac tamponade

            1.   pulsus paradoxus (abnormally large decrease in systolic blood pressure and pulse wave amplitude during inspiration)

            2.   JVD with clear lungs

            3.   narrow pulse pressure (difference between SBP and DBP)

            4.   Decreased CO

            5.   Muffled heart sounds

            6.   For more information on Cardiac Tamponade visit: http://goo.gl/umTsKA

Hypertension

1. Overview

    a.   SBP >140 or >90 DBP based on average of three separate readings

    b.   Classified in stages

        i.   Visit Mayo Clinic for more information on stages: http://goo.gl/icZSxe

2. NCLEX Points
   a. Assessment
      i. past cardiovascular, cerebrovascular, renal, or thyroid disease, diabetes, smoking, alcohol use.
      ii. family history
      iii. referred to as silent killer as asymptomatic until end organ damage occurs
   b. Therapeutic Management
      i. record I&O
      ii. assess for cardiovascular changes
      iii. weight reduction and lifestyle changes
      iv. assess renal and neuro status
      v. Medication therapy
         1. ACE Inhibitors
         2. Beta Blockers
         3. Calcium Channel Blockers
         4. Diuretics
      vi. Lifestyle modifications
         1. Sodium restriction
         2. DASH diet
         3. smoking cessation
      vii. Orthostatic hypotension: rapid drop in SBP of 10-20mmHg in upright position
         1. raise slowly
         2. avoid bathes and strenuous activity after taking medications
      viii. Instruct pt to take medications even if asymptomatic

Cardiomyopathy

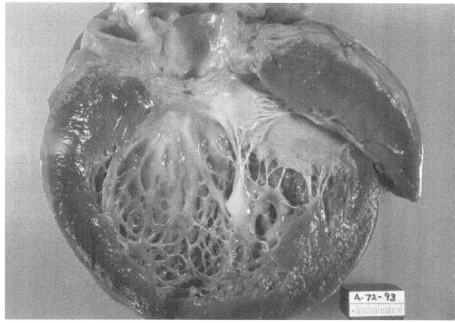

Thickened, dilated left ventricle

1. Overview
    a. Abnormality of heart muscle leading to functional changes
    b. Three types
        i. Dilated: all 4 chambers enlarged, ↓ contractility, ↓CO
        ii. Hypertrophic: progressive thickening of ventricular muscle, ↓CO
        iii. Restrictive: rigid ventricular walls do not stretch during filling, leads to right HF, ↓SV, ↓CO
2. NCLEX® Points
    a. Assessment
        i. fatigue (dyspnea)
        ii. dysrhythmias
        iii. extra heart sounds (s3 and s4)
    b. Therapeutic Management
        i. monitor for signs of HF
        ii. Encourage rest and minimize stress

iii.   Ventricular assistive devices

Peripheral Arterial Disease

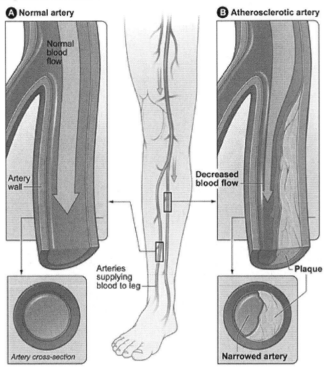

1. Overview
    a. Chronic arterial occlusion leads to decreased oxygen supply to lower extremities
    b. Atherosclerosis most common cause
2. NCLEX® Points
    a. Assessment
        i.   Intermittent claudication (muscle pain following predictable amount of activity relieved by rest)
        ii. Rest pain which awakens the client from sleep
        iii. loss of hair on lower extremities
        iv. Cool, pale, numb extremities

b. Therapeutic Management
    i.   assess pulses
    ii. smoking cessation
    iii. encourage exercise to the point of claudication
         then rest
    iv. Angioplasty
    v.   Endarterectomy
    vi. Bypass grafting

Raynaud's Disease

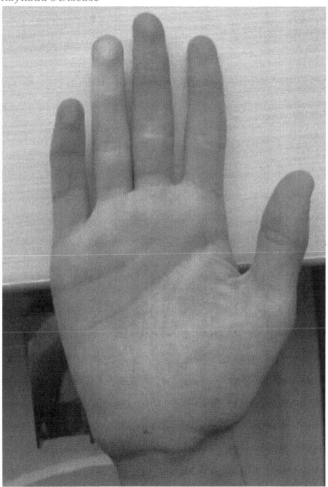

By Thomas Galvin (Own work) [CC BY-SA 4.0
(http://creativecommons.org/licenses/by-sa/4.0)], via Wikimedia Commons

1. Overview
   a. Vasospasm of small arteries and arterioles of hands (less commonly feet, cheeks, ears)
   b. Occur when exposed to cold or stress
2. NCLEX® Points
   a. Assessment
      i. Triphasic color changes (pallor, cyanosis, rubor)
      ii. numbness, tingling, swelling
   b. Therapeutic Management
      i. identify and avoid precipitating factors
      ii. smoking cessation
      iii. wear warm clothing
      iv. medications
         1. analgesics
         2. vasodilators
         3. calcium channel blockers (vasospasm prevention)

Buerger's Disease (thromboangiitis obliterans)
1. Overview
   a. Inflammatory disease of the medium to small arteries and veins of the arms and legs
   b. microthrombi form and lead to vasospasm
2. NCLEX® Points
   a. Assessment
      i. Rest pain
      ii. Intermittent claudication
      iii. pain is most severe at night
      iv. diminished pulses
      v. ulceration in extremities
   b. Therapeutic Management
      i. smoking cessation
      ii. Medication
         1. Calcium channel blockers (prevent vasospasm)
         2. analgesics
      iii. Surgical treatment

1. bypass grafting
2. sympathectomy - surgical dissection of nerve fibers

Aortic Aneurysm

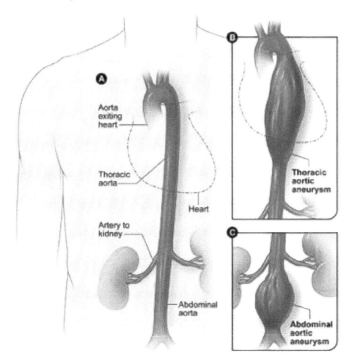

1. Overview
   a. dilation/out pouching of the aorta due to weakened medial layer
   b. classified by location
      i. thoracic
      ii. abdominal
   c. types
      i. dissecting: blood vessels separated by layer of blood
      ii. fusiform: dilation that involves the entire circumference
      iii. saccular: localized out pouching

            iv.   false: clot forms outside the vessel wall
2.   NCLEX® Points
     a.   Assessment
          i.   thoracic
               1.   pain in back, shoulders, abdomen
               2.   dyspnea
          ii.   abdominal
               1.   pulsating mass in the abdomen
               2.   systolic bruit
               3.   tenderness on abdominal palpation
               4.   hematoma on flank
         iii.   Rupture assessment
               1.   severe sudden onset of pain
               2.   pain radiating to flank and groin
               3.   signs of shock
     b.   Therapeutic Management
          i.   Reduce blood pressure
          ii.   diagnose via CT or abdominal ultrasound
         iii.   Abdominal aortic aneurysm resection/EVAR (endovascular aneurysm repair)
               1.   assess peripheral pulses
               2.   monitor renal function (due to blood loss and decreased perfusion)
                   a.   urine output, renal labs
               3.   assess vital signs
               4.   assess incision site

Thrombophlebitis

1.   Overview
     a.   thromubs (clot) formation with associated inflammation
     b.   Virchow's Triad
          i.   Venous stasis
          ii.   Damage to inner lining of vein
         iii.   Hypercoagulability of blood
     c.   Risk for pulmonary embolism if detachment occurs
2.   NCLEX® Points
     a.   Assessment
          i.   Risk factors

        1. history of thrombophlebitis, pelvic surgery, obesity, HF, a-fib, immobility, MI, pregnancy, IV therapy, hypercoagulabiity

  ii. Assessment findings

        1. unilateral edema

        2. pain

        3. warm skin

        4. febrile state

        5. Homan's sign - pain on dorsiflexion of foot

  iii. Therapeutic management

        1. analgesia

        2. ultrasound to confirm finding

        3. monitor respiratory status

            a. report pink sputum, tachypnea, tachycardia, chest pain (signs of pulmonary embolism)

        4. monitor circumference of affected limb

        5. monitor distal pulses

        6. smoking cessation

        7. avoid long periods of sitting

        8. elevate legs 10-20 min every few hours

        9. monitor PT and INR for patients on Coumadin (warfarin)

        10. monitor PTT for patients on Heparin therapy

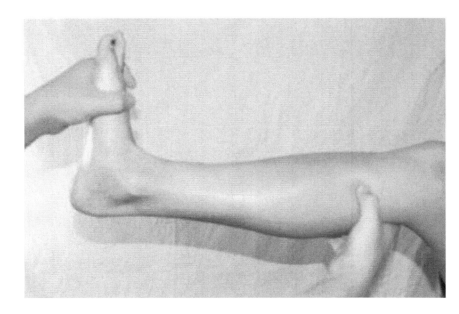

NCLEX® Cram - Cardiovascular

1. Heart Rate
   a. normal sinus 60-100bpm
   b. sinus tachycardia >100bpm
   c. sinus bradycardia <60bpm
2. Vascular System
   a. arteries
      i. carry oxygenated blood to tissues
   b. veins
      i. carry deoxygenated blood back to heart
3. Cardiac Markers
   a. Indication of cardiac damage

Troponin	Most sensitive to cardiac damage	12 hours
CK-MB	Sensitive when skeletal damage isn't present	10-24 hours
Myoglobin (Mb)	Low specificity to infarction	2 hours

4. Labs
   a. Potassium
      i. Hypokalemia
         1. ventricular dysrhythmias
         2. ↑ digoxin toxicity
         3. U wave
         4. ST depression
      ii. Hyperkalemia
         1. Peaked T waves
         2. Wide QRS
         3. Ventricular dysrhythmias
   b. ↑ Hematocrit indicates volume depletion
   c. ↓Hematocrit and hemoglobin indicate anemia
   d. Lipids
      i. Total cholesterol ↓200 mg/dL
      ii. LDL ↓130 mg/dL
      iii. HDL 30-70 mg/dL
5. Holter monitoring provides 24 hour EKG monitoring
   a. client should record any moment that they have chest pain
6. Assess for iodine, seafood allergies prior to any dye tests

7. Cardiac Catheterization
    a. used to assess cardiac function (valve and chamber function)
    b. monitor distal pulses
    c. monitor pressure dressing and insertion site for bleeding or hematoma
8. Angioplasty
    a. used to dilate occluded cardiac vessels
    b. encourage fluid intake to flush dye from system
    c. assess distal pulses
9. Cardioversion
    a. synchronized to R wave
        i. if not synchronized shock could cause VF
10. Coronary artery disease
    a. narrowing of coronary arteries due to plaque build up
        i. may lead to MI, HF, HTN, angina
        ii. ST depression occurs with ischemia
    b. client should follow low fat, low cholesterol, high fiber diet
11. Vena Cava Filter
    a. assess cardiac, neuro, and respiratory status post op
    b. avoid hip flexion
    c. assess for bleeding and hematoma at insertion site
    d. assess peripheral pulses
    e. anti embolic stockings
    f. anti coagulant therapy
12. Cardiogenic Shock
    a. heart is unable maintain effective cardiac output
    b. Assessment
        i. low urine output
        ii. ↓BP
        iii. Assess CVP (pressure in superior vena cava representing right atrial pressure preload)
            1. CVP: 2-8 mmHg
            2. reading should be taken at end expiration if ventilated
            3. Zero transducer at the fourth intercostal space along the mid axillary line (location of the right atrium)

Respiratory Disorders

Asthma

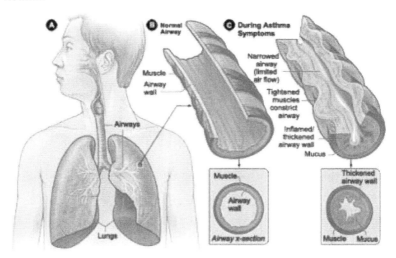

1. Overview
   a. Inflammatory disorder of the airways stimulated by triggers (infection, allergens, exercise, irritant)
   b. Status asthmaticus is a life-threatening condition unresponsive to treatment
2. NCLEX® Points
   a. Assessment
      i. wheezing/crackles
      ii. restlessness
      iii. diminished breath sounds
      iv. tachypnea
   b. Therapeutic Management
      i. High Fowler's position
      ii. Administer O2
      iii. Administer bronchodilators BEFORE corticosteroids

Chronic Obstructive Pulmonary Disease (COPD)

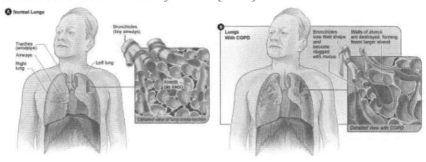

1. Overview
   a. Obstruction of airflow due to emphysema and chronic bronchitis
      i. emphysema
         1. destruction of alveoli due to chronic inflammation
         2. decreased surface area for gas exchange
      ii. chronic bronchitis
         1. chronic airway inflammation with productive cough
         2. excessive sputum production
2. NCLEX® Points
   a. Assessment
      i. Barrel chest
      ii. use of accessory muscles
      iii. congestion on chest Xray
      iv. ABG with $\uparrow CO_2$ and $\downarrow$ pH (respiratory acidosis)
   b. Therapeutic Management
      i. Do not administer O2 at greater than 2 L/min
         1. stimulus to breath is low Po2 not elevated Pco2 (as in healthy individuals)
         2. assess SpO2
         3. provide chest physiotherapy (CPT)
         4. teach pursed lip breathing
         5. avoid allergens and triggers (dust, infections, spicy foods, smoking)

6. Increase fluid intake to 3000 mL/day to keep secretions thin
7. small frequent meals to prevent hypoxia

Pneumothorax and Hemothorax

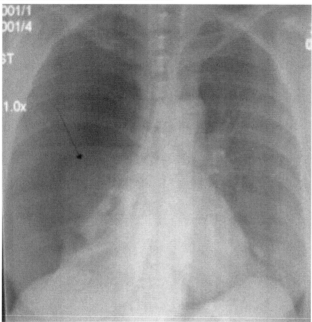

1. Overview
    a. Pneumothorax
        i.   Spontaneous: ruptured bleb on lung surface fills pleural space compressing lung (collapsed lung)
             1. primary: rupture of bleb in otherwise healthy individual
             2. secondary: rupture of distended alveoli may occur with COPD
        ii. Tension: injury to chest wall leading to shift in mediastinum to unaffected side and disruption of venous return to the heart. This is a medical emergency due to severely compromised cardiac output and building pressure in chest cavity.
    b. Hemothorax

          i.   Blood accumulation in pleural space

2.   NCLEX® Points

    a.   Assessment

        i.   Decreased or absent breath sounds on affected side

        ii.   decreased chest expansion on affected side

        iii.   tracheal deviation to unaffected side (tension pneumothorax)

        iv.   Dullness (hemothorax)

        v.   dyspnea

        vi.   hyperresonance (pneumothorax)

    b.   Therapeutic Management

        i.   chest tube insertion

        ii.   thoracentesis

        iii.   high Fowler's position

        iv.   Open pneumothorax

            1.   if the pneumothorax is due to an open (sucking) chest wound the hole should be covered immediately with a nonporous (occlusive) dressing sealed on three sides. This prevents air from entering during inhalation while allowing it to escape during expiration.

Pneumonia

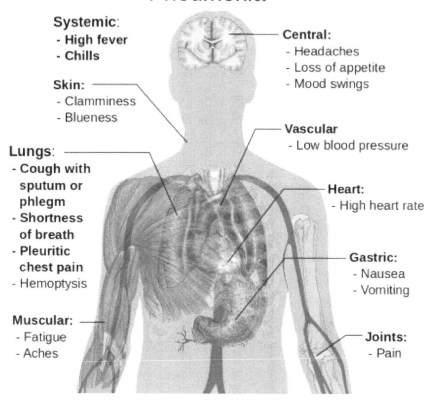

Main symptoms of infectious
Pneumonia

Systemic:
- High fever
- Chills

Skin:
- Clamminess
- Blueness

Central:
- Headaches
- Loss of appetite
- Mood swings

Vascular
- Low blood pressure

Lungs:
- Cough with sputum or phlegm
- Shortness of breath
- Pleuritic chest pain
- Hemoptysis

Heart:
- High heart rate

Gastric:
- Nausea
- Vomiting

Muscular:
- Fatigue
- Aches

Joints:
- Pain

1. Overview
    a. Inflammatory condition of the lungs primarily affecting the alveoli which may fill with fluid or pus.
    b. Infectious vs Noninfectious
        i. infectious
            1. bacterial vs viral
        ii. non infectious
            1. aspiration
    c. Community acquired vs Hospital acquired vs Opportunistic
    d. Chest Xray and Sputum culture necessary
    e. sputum culture identifies organism
2. NCLEX® Points

a. Assessment
   i. Viral
     1. low grade fever
     2. non productive cough
     3. WBCs normal to low elevation
     4. Chest X-ray shows minimal changes
     5. less severe than bacterial
   ii. Bacterial
     1. high fever
     2. productive cough
     3. WBCs elevated
     4. Chest X-ray shows infiltrates
     5. more severe
b. NCLEX® Points
   i. Assessment
     1. As above
     2. chills
     3. rhonchi and wheezes
     4. sputum production
   ii. Therapeutic Management
     1. antibiotics, analgesics, antipyretics
     2. supplemental O2
     3. maintain airway and assess respiratory status
     4. encourage activity as soon as possible
     5. instruct on chest expansion exercises, coughing and deep breathing
     6. obtain vaccinations for influenza and pneumococcal pneumonia
     7. proper hand hygiene
     8. encourage 3 L/day of fluids unless contraindicated

Tuberculosis
1. Overview
a. Lung infection causing pneumonitis and granulomas in the lungs
b. Noncompliance with treatment may lead to drug resistance (MDR-TB)
c. Transmission caused by airborn route via droplets

2. NCLEX® Points
   a. When contact with an infected individual occurs chest x-ray and skin test are completed
   b. Risk of transmission is reduced after 2-3 weeks of medication regimen
   c. Assessment
      i. Night sweets
      ii. Chills
      iii. Fatigue
      iv. Weight loss
      v. Persistent cough
   d. Client history
      i. Foreign travel
      ii. Living in tight quarters
      iii. Past exposure
      iv. Sputum cultures
   e. Therapeutic Management
      i. Place in a negative pressure room
      ii. Skin test should be measured in size
      iii. Particulate respirator must be worn
      iv. Isoniazide, pyrazinamide and rifampin
      v. Treatment should continue for 6-12 months

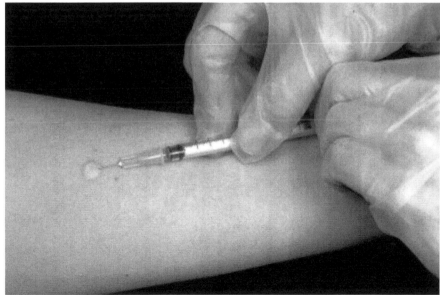

Pulmonary Embolism (PE)

1. Overview
    a. Emboli in pulmonary circulation block blood flow to pulmonary capillaries
    b. Common causes
        i. immobilization
        ii. long bone fractures
        iii. hypercoagulabiity
        iv. DVT in large veins
    c. Gas exchange is impaired leading to pulmonary infarction
2. NCLEX® Points
    a. Assessment
        i. VQ scan (ventilation perfusion scan) used to diagnose
        ii. Low PaO2
        iii. restlessness, anxiety
        iv. Tachycardia, tachypnea, hypotension, fever
        v. Altered LOC
        vi. diaphoresis and cyanosis
    b. Therapeutic Management
        i. O2 therapy
        ii. prepare for ventilation
        iii. Anticoagulant
        iv. Analgesics
        v. Vena cava filter insertion

NCLEX® Cram - Respiratory

1. Sputum culture
    a. obtain sample prior to beginning antibiotic therapy
2. Keep client NPO post bronchoscopy until gag reflex returns
3. Thoracentesis

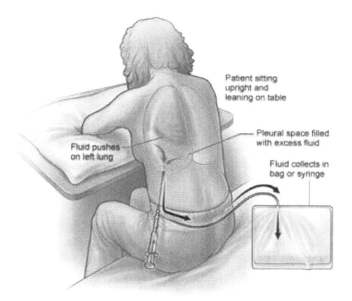

- a. position the client sitting upright leaning forward onto a bedside table with arms supporting weight
- b. monitor for pneumothorax and PE

4. Lung Biopsy - Post Procedure
- a. monitor sight for drainage and bleeding
- b. monitor respiratory status and assess for signs of pneumothorax

5. Normal ABG Values
- a. pH: 7.35 - 7.45
- b. PCO2: 35-45 mmHg
- c. HCO3: 22-26 mEq/L
- d. PO2: 80-100 mmHg
- e. SpO2: 96%-100%
- f. Acedemia = pH <7.35
- g. Alkalemia = pH>7.45

6. SpO2: % of O2 bound to hemoglobin compared to total HgB capable of binding)
- a. remove nail polish
- b. poor circulation will diminish accuracy

7. Hierarchy of O2 Delivery

Method
Nasal Cannula
1 lpm = 24%
2 lpm = 28%
3 lpm = 32%
4 lpm = 36%
5 lpm = 40%
6 lpm = 44%
Simple Face Mask
5 lpm = 40%
6 lpm = 45-50%
7 lpm = 50-55%
8 lpm = 55-60%
Non-rebreather Mask
6 lpm = 60%
7 lpm = 70%
8 lpm = 80%
9 lpm = 90%
10 lpm = close to 100%
Venturi Mask
4 lpm = 24-28%
8 lpm = 35-40%
12 lpm = 50%
Trach Collar
21-70% at 10L
T-Piece
21-100% with flow rate at 2.5 times minute ventilation
CPAP
Positive airway pressure during spontaneous breaths
Bi-PAP
Positive pressure during spontaneous breaths (IPAP) and preset pressure to be maintained during expiration (EPAP/PEEP)
SIMV
Preset Vt and f. Circuit remains open between mandatory breaths so pt can take additional breaths. Ventilator doesn't cycle during spontaneous breaths so Vt varies.

Mandatory breaths synchronized so they do not occur during spontaneous breaths.
Assist Control **Preset Vt and f and inspiratory effort required to assist spontaneous breaths.** **Delivers control breaths. Cycles additionally if pt inspiratory effort is adequate.** **Same Vt delivered for spontaneous breaths.**

7. Ventilator Alarms
   a. High Pressure
      i. Kink in tubing
      ii. cough, gag, or biting tube
      iii. increased secretions
   b. Low Pressure
      i. ET tube disconnection
8. Rib fractures will cause pain during inspiration
9. Flail chest causes paradoxical respirations
10. Acute Respiratory Distress Syndrome (ARDS)
    a. ABG: respiratory acidosis (pH<7.35 CO2>45 PaO2 <80)
11. Tripod position and pursed lipped breathing helpful to COPD patients
12. Influenza
    a. vaccination recommended yearly for
       i. health care workers
       ii. elderly
       iii. children
       iv. immunocompromised
13. If a patient has an injured neck use chin thrust rather than head tilt to open airway
14. Limit airway suctioning to 10 seconds
15. Rotate catheter and use intermittent suction
16. Lung injury - Good Lung Down positioning
17. High fowlers (>45 degrees) positioning for respiratory failure patients
18. Mask should be worn at all times with droplet isolation
19. Pink Puffer vs Blue Bloater
    a. Pink Puffer: emphysema
       i. barrel-shaped chest, hyperinflated chest, pursed lipped breathing

b. Blue Bloater: bronchitis
   i. hypoxia, obese, water retention, dependent on hypoxia for respiratory drive
20. Atelectisis: incomplete expansion or collapse of lung

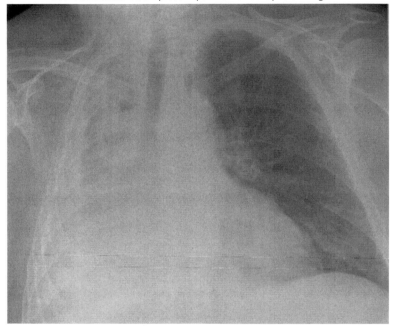

By The original uploader was Pabloes at Spanish Wikipedia (Transferred from es.wikipedia to Commons.) [GFDL (http://www.gnu.org/copyleft/fdl.html) or CC-BY-SA-3.0 (http://creativecommons.org/licenses/by-sa/3.0/)], via Wikimedia Commons

Neurological Disorders

Increased Intracranial Pressure (ICP)

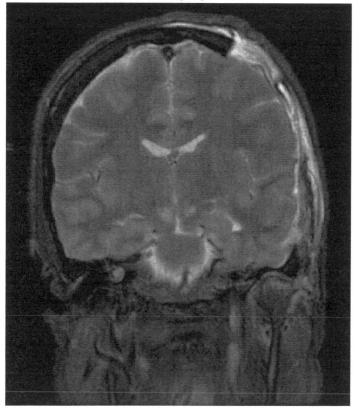

By Rocque BG, Başkaya MK [CC BY 2.0
(http://creativecommons.org/licenses/by/2.0)], via Wikimedia Commons

Increasing ICP can lead to brain herniation

1. Overview
    a. Normal ICP: 5-15mmHg
    b. ICP can elevate due to trauma, hemorrhage, tumor,
        hydrocephlaus, inflammation

      c.   The cranial vault is rigid, increased ICP can limit cerebral perfusion, impeded CSF absorption and lead to herniation of brain tissue causing death

  2.   NCLEX® Points

      a.   Assessment

           i.   Levels of Consciousness

Conscious	Normal	Assessment of LOC involves checking orientation: people who are able promptly and spontaneously to state their name, location, and the date or time are said to be oriented to self, place, and time, or "oriented X3". A normal sleep stage from which a person is easily awakened is also considered a normal level of consciousness. "Clouding of consciousness" is a term for a mild alteration of consciousness with alterations in attention and wakefulness.
Confused	Disoriented; impaired thinking and responses	People who do not respond quickly with information about their name, location, and the time are considered "obtuse" or "confused". A confused person may be bewildered, disoriented, and have difficulty following instructions. The person may have slow thinking and possible memory time loss. This could be caused by sleep deprivation, malnutrition, allergies, environmental pollution, drugs (prescription and nonprescription), and infection.
Delirious	Disoriented; restlessness, hallucinations, sometimes delusions	Some scales have "delirious" below this level, in which a person may be restless or agitated and exhibit a marked deficit in attention.
Somnolent	Sleepy	A *somnolent* person shows excessive drowsiness and responds to stimuli only with incoherent mumbles or disorganized movements.
Obtunded	Decreased alertness; slowed psychomotor responses	In *obtundation*, a person has a decreased interest in their surroundings, slowed responses, and sleepiness.

Stuporous	Sleep-like state (not unconscious); little/no spontaneous activity	People with an even lower level of consciousness, stupor, only respond by grimacing or drawing away from painful stimuli.
Comatose	Cannot be aroused; no response to stimuli	Cannot be aroused; no response to stimuli

      ii.   headache
      iii. Cushing's Triad
           1.   abnormal respirations
           2.   widening pulse pressure
           3.   reflex bradycardia
      iv. elevated temp
      v.   pupilary changes
      vi. posturing
      vii. seizures
      viii. positive Babinski reflex
   b.   Therapeutic Management
      i.   monitory respiratory status
      ii.   monitor pupil changes
      iii. avoid sedatives and CNS depressants
      iv. Hypocapnia (PaCO2 30-35 mmHg) will lead to cerebral vasoconstriction leading to decreased ICP
      v.   monitor temperature
      vi. prevent shivering
      vii. decrease stimuli
      viii. monitor electrolytes
      ix. avoid Valsalva's maneuver
      x.   Ventricular drain and ICP monitoring
      xi. Assess neuro status q 1-2 hours
      xii. elevate HOB to at least 30 degrees
      xiii. Osmotic diuretics and corticosteroids

Stroke

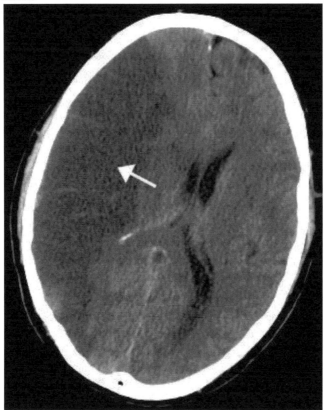

By INFARCT.jpg: Lucien Monfils derivative work: Suraj (INFARCT.jpg) [CC BY-SA 3.0 (http://creativecommons.org/licenses/by-sa/3.0) or GFDL (http://www.gnu.org/copyleft/fdl.html)], via Wikimedia Commons

Right MCA Infarct

1. Overview
    a. Neurological deficit caused by decreased blood flow to a portion of the brain
    b. May be ischemic or hemorrhagic
    c. Lack of blood flow greater than 10 minutes can cause irreversible damage
    d. Risk factors:

          i.   HTN

          ii.   Diabetes

          iii.   atherosclerosis

          iv.   cardiac dysrhythmias

          v.   substance abuse

          vi.   obesity

          vii.   oral contraceptives

          viii.   anticoagulant therapy

    e.   Diagnosed via: CT, MRI, cerebral arteriogram (hemorrhagic and late ischemic)

2.   NCLEX® Points

    a.   Assessment

          i.   contralateral manifestations (opposite side of stroke)

          ii.   FAST

                1.   facial droop

                2.   arms - does one arm drift?

                3.   speech problems

                4.   time - call 9-1-1

          iii.   dependent on location

                1.   Aphasia   - speech difficulty

                    a.   Expressive - understands but unable to communicate verbally

                    b.   Receptive - unable to comprehend spoke and written word

                    c.   Global - language dysfunction

                    d.   Interventions

                          i.   provide adequate time for client to respond

                          ii.   repeat names of individuals and objects frequently

                          iii.   use a picture board

        iv.   provide only one instruction at a time
2. Apraxia - inability to perform tasks
3. Hemianopsia - blindness in half the vision field
      a. instruct client to turn head to capture the entire vision field
      b. approach client from unaffected side
      c. provide food and objects to unaffected side
4. Dysphagia - difficulty swallowing
b. Therapeutic Management
   i. involve speech therapy
   ii. ischemic stroke
      1. permissive hypertension
      2. antithrombitic therapy
      3. carotid endartecomy
      4. thrombectomy
      5. monitor neurological status
   iii. hemorrhagic stroke
      1. coiling or clipping of aneurysm
      2. monitor neurological status
   iv. seizure precautions
   v. monitor level of consciousness
   vi. monitor neurological status
   vii. maintain quiet, calm environment
   viii. assess need for assistive devices
   ix. involve physical and occupational therapy

Seizure Disorder

View the NRSNG.com video on Seizures here: https://youtu.be/lr2G34fl4Fg

1. Overview
    a. Abnormal excessive discharge of electrical activity in the brain
    b. Types
        i. Generalized - both hemispheres
            1. Tonic-clonic
            2. absence
            3. myoclonic
            4. atonic
        ii. Partial - one hemisphere
            1. simple partial
            2. complex partial
    c. Risk factors
        i. genetics
        ii. trauma
        iii. tumors
        iv. toxicity
        v. infection
        vi. cerebral bleeding or swelling
        vii. acute febrile state
    d. Status epilepticus - persistent seizure activity with little or no break
2. NCLEX® Points
    a. Assessment
        i. assess for Aura (sensation that warns of impending seizure)
        ii. Postictal state (period after seizure): memory loss, sleepiness, impaired speech
        iii. assess type, onset, duration
    b. Therapeutic Management
        i. Maintain patent airway
            1. turn client to side
            2. have O2 and suction equipment available after the seizure

                    3. DO NOT force anything into the mouth during the seizure (including bite block)
- ii. prevent injury
    1. bed to the lowest position
    2. padded side rails
    3. loosen restrictive clothing
    4. DO NOT try to restrain client
- iii. Document onset, preceding events, duration, and postictal events
- iv. Medications
    1. Anitepileptics
    2. Diazepam, Lorazepam, phenobarbital are often given during seizure activity
- v. Educate client and family on importance of medication compliance
- vi. Educate family on care during seizure

Parkinson's Disease

1. Overview
   a. Degenerative neurological disorder caused by atrophy of substantia negra leading to depletion of dopamine. This leads to termination of acetylcholine inhibition which causes symptoms.
   b. Dopamine plays a role in the inhibition of excitatory impulses. When this neurotransmitter is depleted acetylcholine is no longer inhibited.
   c. Slow, progressive disease.
   d. client becomes progressively debilitated and self-care dependent
2. NCLEX® Points
   a. Assessment
      i. bradykinesia: slow movements due to muscle rigidity
      ii. resting tremor
      iii. Pill rolling - tremors in hands and fingers
      iv. Akinesia
      v. blank facial expression
      vi. shuffling steps, stooped stance, drooling

     vii. dysphagia
  b. Therapeutic Management
     i. Assistive devices
     ii. involvement of speech, physical, and occupational therapy
     iii. monitor diet to insure proper caloric intake
       1. increase fluid intake
       2. high protein
       3. high fiber
     iv. Assess ability to swallow prior to anything by mouth
     v. Use rocking movement to initiate movement
     vi. encourage client to ambulate multiple times a day
     vii. participate in active and passive range of motion activities
     viii. avoid foods high in Vitamin B6 (blocks effects of antiparkinsonian drugs)
     ix. small, frequent, nutrient dense foods
     x. Medication therapy
       1. dopaminergics, dopamine agonists, anticholinergics
       2. goal is to increase the level of dopamine in the CNS
       3. eventually drugs become ineffective

Multiple Sclerosis

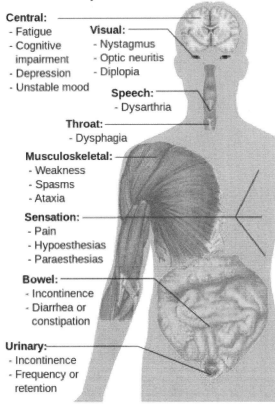

Main symptoms of
Multiple sclerosis

Central:
- Fatigue
- Cognitive impairment
- Depression
- Unstable mood

Visual:
- Nystagmus
- Optic neuritis
- Diplopia

Speech:
- Dysarthria

Throat:
- Dysphagia

Musculoskeletal:
- Weakness
- Spasms
- Ataxia

Sensation:
- Pain
- Hypoesthesias
- Paraesthesias

Bowel:
- Incontinence
- Diarrhea or constipation

Urinary:
- Incontinence
- Frequency or retention

1. Overview
   a. Chronic, progressive demyelinization of the neurons in the CNS
   b. Remission and exacerbation
   c. Primarily ages 20-40 years old
2. NCLEX® Points
   a. Assessment
      i. fatigue
      ii. tremors
      iii. spasticity of muscles
      iv. bladder dysfunction

     v. decrease peripheral sensation (pain, temperature, touch)
     vi. visual disturbances
     vii. emotional instability
   b. Therapeutic Management
     i. No cure - supportive therapy
     ii. energy conservation
     iii. maintain adequate fluid intake 2000 mL/day
     iv. provide bowel and bladder training
     v. encourage activity independence
     vi. regulate temperatures on water heaters, baths, and heating pads
     vii. insure in home safety (rugs, cords, etc)

Myasthenia Gravis

1. Overview
  a. Chronic progressive disorder of the PNS which affects transmission of nerve impulses
  b. Onset often caused by precipitating factors (stress, hormone disturbance, infection, trauma, temperature)
  c. Insufficient secretion of acetylcholine with excessive secretion of cholinesterase
2. NCLEX® Points
  a. Assessment
    i. weakness/fatigue
    ii. diplopia (double vision) and ptosis (drooping eyelid)

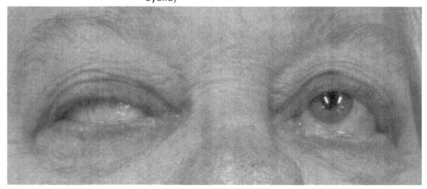

By James Heilman, MD (Own work) [CC BY-SA 3.0 (http://creativecommons.org/licenses/by-sa/3.0)], via Wikimedia Commons

   iii. monitor respiratory status
- 1. swallowing, respirations, tachypnea, abnormal ABG, breath sounds, difficulty breathing

   iv. Cholinergic crisis: severe muscle weakness due to overmedication; cramps, diarrhea, bradycardia, bronchial spasm
- 1. Assessment
  - a. N/V, diarrhea
  - b. hypotension
  - c. blurred vision
- 2. Intervention
  - a. withhold medication
  - b. administer antidote

   v. Myasthenic crisis: acute exacerbation of disease, sudden severe motor weakness, risk of respiratory failure, caused by insufficient medication dosage
- 1. Assessment
  - a. increase pulse, respirations, bp
  - b. anoxia and cyanosis
  - c. bowel and bladder dysfunction
- 2. Intervention
  - a. increase medication

   vi. Tensilon test
- 1. used to confirm diagnosis
  - a. client at risk of vfib and cardiac arrest have atropine available

b. Therapeutic Management
   i. monitor respiratory status
   ii. maintain suction and emergency equipment
   iii. insure proper medication
   iv. monitor feeding and insure proper nutrition

1. schedule medication 30-40 minutes prior to meals
   v. provide adequate eye care
   vi. instruct client to avoid temperature extremes, emotional stress, drugs, alcohol, and exposure to infection
   vii. educate on signs of cholinergic and myasthenic crisis

NCLEX® Cram - Neurological Disorders

1. Glasgow Coma Scale

Score	1	2	3	4	5	6
Eyes	Does not open	Opens to painful stimuli	Opens to voice	Opens spontaneously	N/A	N/A
Verbal	Makes no sound	Incomprehensible sounds	Utters inappropriate words	Confused, disoriented	Oriented, converses normally	N/A
Motor	Makes no movements	Extension to painful stimuli	Flexion to painful stimuli	Withdraws to painful stimuli	Localizes to pain	Obeys commands

2. Hypothalamus
   a. regulates body temperature
   b. regulates response to sympathetic and parasympathetic nervous system
   c. produces hormones secreted by pituitary gland and hypothalamus
3. Pons
   a. regulates breathing

4. CT Scan

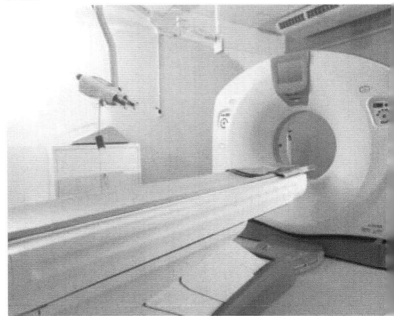

    a. assess for allergy to contrast, shellfish, iodine if dye is used

    b. provide adequate fluids to flush dye if used

5. MRI

    a. remove all metal objects from patients

    b. determine if client has a pacemaker - cannot complete MRI with pacemaker

6. Cerebral Angiography

    a. assess for allergies to dye

    b. maintain flat bed rest or at the position the physician orders

    c. assess insertion site for swelling, hematoma, and bleeding

7. Level of consciousness is the most essential indicator of neurological status

8. Pupil Assessment

    a. Pupils equal and react to light

    b. Pupil reacts slowly to light

    c. Dilated pupil (compressed cranial nerve III)

    d. Bilateral pupilary dilation, fixed (ominous)

    e. Bilateral pinpoint (pons damage)

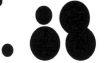

9. Client position
   a. Decorticate
      i. flexes both arms on chest (toward CORd)
      ii. cortex damage

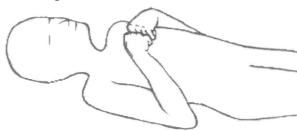

   b. Decerebrate
      i. extends arms and/or legs
      ii. brainstem lesion
   c. Flaccid
      i. no motor response to stimuli
10. Babinski test
    a. dorsiflexion of the big toe indicating neurologic damage

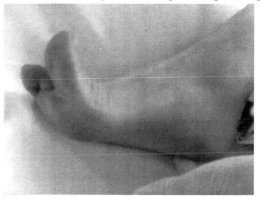

11. Hyperthermia can increase cerebral O2 demands and lead to hypoxia
    a. initiate seizure precautions
12. Halo Sign
    a. CSF will separate from blood when placed on a white sterile background
13. Do not suction or blow nose with traumatic head injury or pituitary surgery

14. Diabetes insipidus results from inadequate secretion of ADH and can be manifested as copious amounts of urine output. This reflects damage to the pituitary gland.
15. Immobilize clients when spinal injury is suspected
16. Clean pin sites on halo traction devices daily
    a. Do not shower
    b. keep pin sites clean, assess skin, report any redness or swelling
17. Turn spinal patients using the log rolling technique
18. Trigeminal Neuralgia
    a. damage to fifth cranial nerve
    b. severe pain to cheeks, lips, gums
    c. extreme temperatures may exacerbate symptoms
    d. client should avoid hot or cold foods and fluids
19. Bell's Palsy
    a. sudden weakness in the muscles on one half of face
    b. usually resolves within 6 months without treatment
    c. steroids and antivirals may be provided
    d. protect eyes from dryness
    e. chew food on unaffected side

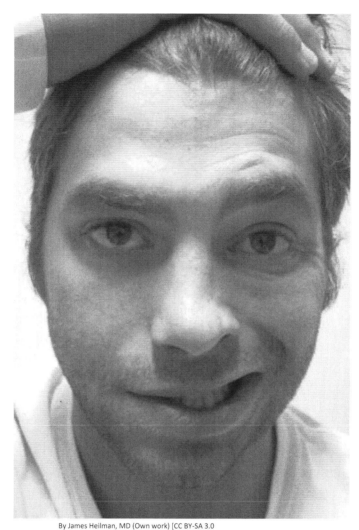

By James Heilman, MD (Own work) [CC BY-SA 3.0
(http://creativecommons.org/licenses/by-sa/3.0) or GFDL
(http://www.gnu.org/copyleft/fdl.html)], via Wikimedia Commons

20. Guillain-Barre Syndrome

  a. monitor respiratory status closely

21. West Nile Virus

  a. symptoms develop 3-14 days after being bitten by infected
      mosquito

  b. fever, headache, tremors, seizures, coma, vision loss

  c. DEET bug spray should be worn

22. Meningitis
   a. inflammation of the brain and spinal cord membranes due to infection by virus, bacteria, or fungus, protozoa

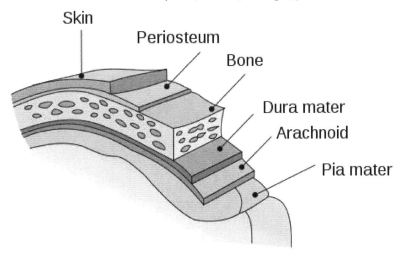

   b. CSF is analyzed to determine diagnosis
       i. cloudy, ↑WBC, ↓Glucose
   c. Nuchal rigidity
   d. photophobia
   e. lethargy
   f. altered level of consciousness
   g. positive Kernig and Burdzinski's sign
   h. client should be placed in isolation
   i. administer analgesics and antibiotics
   j. initiate seizure precautions
   k. Assess for ↑ICP
   l. Transmission usually occurs in areas of population density and crowded living spaces

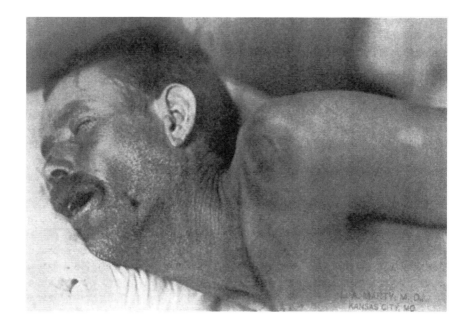

Renal and Genitourinary Disorders

Acute Kidney Injury

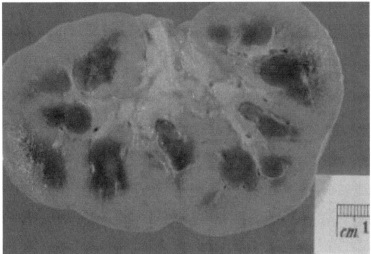

Damaged kidney

1. Overview
    a. Sudden loss of renal function due to poor circulation or renal cell damage
    b. usually reversible may resolve on its own, can lead to permanent damage if not reversed quickly
    c. Causes
        i. Prerenal: decreased blood flow to kidneys, accounts for majority of cases
        ii. Intrarenal: within the kidney due to tubular necrosis, infection, obstruction, prolonged ischemia
        iii. Postrenal: damage between the kidney and urethral meatus generally caused by infection, calculi, obstruction
    d. Phases
        i. Progresses in phases
            1. Onset
            2. Oliguric

        a. decreased urine output <400 mL/day

        b. signs of hypervolemia (HTN, HF, edema, pericardial effusion)

        c. pericarditis

        d. Therapeutic Management

          i. restrict fluid intake

          ii. identify cause

          iii. diuretics

3. Diuretic

        a. gradual urine output increase followed by diuresis

        b. Therapeutic Management

          i. replace fluids and electrolytes

4. Recovery

    ii. Can progress to chronic kidney injury if not reversed

    iii. Signs and symptoms result from kidneys inability to regulate fluid and electrolytes

2. NCLEX® Points

    a. Assessment

      i. Azotemia (retention of nitrogen waste in blood)

      ii. monitor urine output

      iii. monitor weight daily

      iv. monitor for infection

      v. monitor for fluid overload (edema, crackles, wheezes)

      vi. monitor for metabolic acidosis

      vii. prepare for dialysis

Chronic Kidney Disease

1. Overview

    a. Progressive, irreversible loss of renal function with associated decline in GFR

    b. all body systems affected dialysis is required

    c. ESRD occurs with GFR <15mL/min

    d. Causes

    i. DM

    ii. HTN

    iii. unreversed AKI

    iv. glomerulonephritis

    v. autoimmune disorders

2. NCLEX® Points

  a. Assessment

    i. azotemia

    ii. ↑BUN, creatinine

    iii. Cardio

      1. HTN, hypervolemia, CHF

    iv. Hematologic

      1. anemia

      2. thrombocytopenia

    v. Gastrointestinal

      1. anorexia

      2. N/V

    vi. Neurological

      1. lethargy

      2. confusion

      3. coma

    vii. Urinary

      1. ↓ urine output

      2. proteinuria

    viii. Skeletal

      1. osteoporosis

  b. Therapeutic Management

    i. epoetin alfa aids in countering anemia

    ii. avoid administering asprin

    iii. monitor potassium levles

      1. ↑ potassium can lead to EKG changes (peaked T waves, flat P, wide QRS, blocks, asystole)

      2. provide low potassium diet

      3. Potassium lowering medications

        a. Kayexalate

        b. insulin

        c. calcium gluconate

      4. provide continuous cardiac monitoring

iv. phosphate binders may be required to lower phosphorus levels

v. monitor daily weights

vi. monitor for signs of heart failure

vii. monitor electrolyte levels and BUN Creatinine

viii. assess peripheral nerve function and monitor for peripheral neuropathy

ix. vision can be affected: monitor and provide for a safe environment

x. instruct client on dialysis and provide end of life care as needed

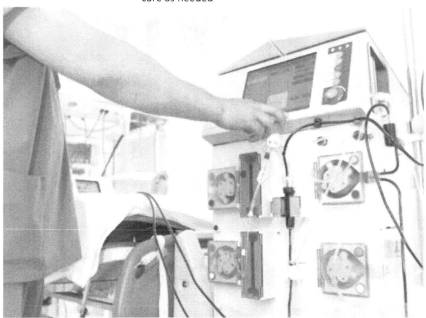

Renal Calculi

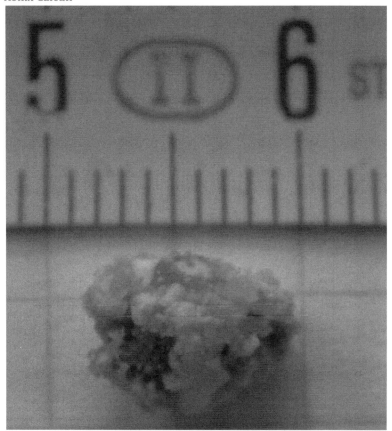

1. Overview
    a. Stones that form in the urinary tract
    b. Form as a result of chemicals in urine becoming concentrated (calcium or oxalate, struvite, uric acid, cystine)
    c. Causes
        i. diet high in calcium, Vit D, protein, purines
        ii. dehydration
        iii. immobilization
        iv. ↑uric acid (gout)
        v. infection
        vi. obstruction

2. NCLEX® Points
   a. Assessment
      i. pain which radiates from lumbar to side to testicles or bladder
      ii. severe pain with sudden onset
      iii. dull pain in renal area
      iv. signs of UTI
      v. hematuria (blood in urine)
   b. Therapeutic Management
      i. monitor VS looking for infection
      ii. increase fluid intake to 3000 mL/day
      iii. provide analgesia to treat pain
      iv. promote ambulation
      v. strain all urine to catch stone
      vi. Treatment options
         1. Extracoporeal Shock-wave Lithotripsy (ESWL)
            a. external shock waves generated to pulverize stone
         2. Lithotomy
            a. surgical removal
         3. Nephrostomy
            a. small flank incision with stone removal via endoscope
         4. Uroscopy
            a. urethral catheter inserted via cystoscope

Glomerulonephritis
1. Overview
   a. Inflammatory disorder of the glomerulus caused by immunological reaction
   b. Predisposing factors
      i. upper respiratory infection
      ii. skin infection
      iii. SLE
2. NCLEX® Points
   a. Assessment
      i. fever

      ii.   anorexia, N/V

      iii. malaise

      iv. ↑BUN and Creatinine, ↓Creatinine clearance

      v.   ↓ uptake and excretion of dye with renal scan

      vi. HTN

      vii. Hypoalbuminemia

      viii. hematuria, protneinuria

b. Therapeutic Management

      i.   Plasmapheresis: removal of harmful antibodies from plasma

      ii. dialysis

      iii. protein restriction, ↓K+, ↓Na+

      iv. bedrest

      v.   monitor daily weight and I&O

Nephrotic Syndrome

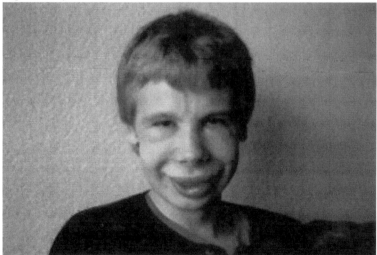

Facial edema from sodium and water retention caused by nephrotic syndrome

1. Overview

   a. Kidney disease characterized by loss of protein from plasma into urine

   b. proteinurea, hypoalbuminemia, edema

   c. Plasma proteins leak into the urine, fluid shift occurs leading to massive edema

2. NCLEX® Points
    a. Assessment
        i.   severe edema
        ii. weight gain
        iii. renal failure symptoms
        iv. fatigue
        v.   amenorrhea
        vi. positive renal biopsy
    b. Therapeutic Management
        i.   goal is to reduce urinary protein excretion,
             reduce edema, minimize further complications
        ii. ↓Na in diet
        iii. high protein diet
        iv. bed rest
        v.   monitor immunologic function
            1. assess for infection
            2. Monitor CBC with attention on WBC
                and differential
            3. hand hygiene

Urinary Tract Infection (UTI)

1. Overview
   a. infection within the urinary tract leading to inflammation
   b. urinary tract is sterile above the urethra, pathogens gain entrance via perineal area or via bloodstream
   c. females are more prone due to shorter urethra
   d. males become more susceptible with age due to urinary stasis
2. NCLEX® Points
   a. Assessment
      i. Urine
         1. cloudy, frequent, strong odor, burning, frequent
      ii. **Confusion (altered mental status) and lethargy in older adults**
      iii. ↑WBCs
      iv. urine cultures reveal bacteria
   b. Therapeutic Management
      i. ↑fluid intake (3000 mL/day)
      ii. antimicrobials
      iii. urine cultures
      iv. antimicrobials, antispasmodics, analgesics
      v. Client education
         1. avoid caffeine, carbonation, alcohol
         2. complete the course of antibiotics
         3. ↑fluid intake
         4. avoid powder, sprays, avoid baths
         5. frequent urination
         6. drink cranberry juice

Benign Prostatic Hyperplasia (BPH)

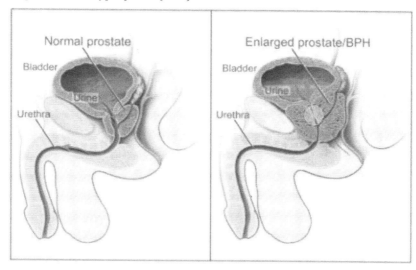

1. Overview
   a. enlargement of the prostate gland leading to partial or total obstruction of the urethra
2. NCLEX® Points
   a. Assessment
      i. feeling of incomplete bladder emptying
      ii. ↓force of urine stream
      iii. nocturia
      iv. postvoid dribbling
      v. urinary stasis
      vi. UTIs
      vii. hematuria
   b. Therapeutic Management
      i. ↑ fluid intake (3000mL/day)
      ii. avoid anything that leads to urinary retention
      iii. follow medication regimen
      iv. create and follow voiding schedule
      v. ↓caffeine, artificial sweeteners, spicy and acidic foods
      vi. TURP - transurethral resection of the prostate

NCLEX® Cram - Renal and Urinary System Disorders

1. Hemodialysis
    a. process of cleaning the blood of waste and toxins by diffusion across a semipermeable membrane
    b. cleanses the clients blood
    c. removes urea, creatinine, uric acid
    d. monitor vital signs closely throughout
    e. monitor labs values closely
    f. weigh the client before and after dialysis to estimate fluid loss
    g. assess for bleeding
    h. hold antihypertensives and medications that might affect blood pressure
    i. hold medications that will be removed by dialysis (contact pharmacy with questions)
    j. Do not use hemodialysis access catheters for anything other than hemodialysis
    k. do not insert IVs on extremity with active shunt
    l. do not assess blood pressure on affected extremity
    m. assess capillary refill in affected extremity
    n. monitor fistulas and grafts closely for clots
        i. Bruit: listen
        ii. Thrill: feel
        iii. Always assess for a bruit and thrill with ESRD patients. If bruit and thrill are absent notify the physician.
    o. complication with dialysis are severe (air embolus, electrolyte imbalance, shock, hemorrhage, sepsis, encephalopathy)
        i. monitor and assess the client thoroughly and frequently
2. Peritoneal Dialysis

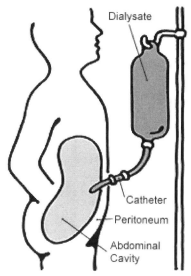

a. peritoneum acts as semipermeable membrane
  i. contraindications
    1. peritonitis
    2. abdominal surgery
  ii. can be continuous (24/7)
b. complications
  i. peritonitis (infection of the peritoneum)
  ii. **cloudy outflow** sign of peritonitis and should be reported
  iii. avoid infection via strict sterile technique

3. Function of the kidneys
  a. maintain acid-base balance
  b. fluid and electrolyte balance
  c. secrete renin to aid in blood pressure regulation and erythropoietin (stimulate bone marrow to produce RBCs)
  d. urine production

4. Creatinine clearance used to estimate GFR (normal 125 mL/minute, decreases with age)

5. Assess allergy to dye, shellfish, iodine prior to urography
  a. instruct to drink fluids to flush dye post procedure unless contraindicated
  b. dye damaging to kidneys

6. Cystoscopy used to examine bladder and take biopsy:
   https://youtu.be/d9Vx3Lgz4sw
7. Renal biopsy
   a. assess coagulation studies
   b. assess client for bleeding from site post procedure
   c. apply pressure to site
8. Urosepsis
   a. most common cause is a urinary catheter
9. Hydronephrosis
   a. renal distention caused by obstruction of normal urine flow
      i. monitor fluid and electrolyte balance

Gastrointestinal Disorders

Gastroesophageal Reflux Disease (GERD)

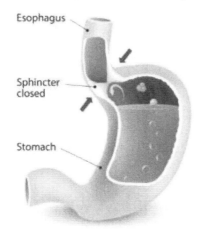
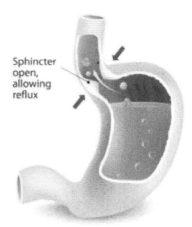

Healthy   **GERD**

1. Overview
   a. Backward movement of gastric contents into esophagus
   b. Due to relaxation of or incompetent lower esophageal sphincter, pyloric stenosis, increased gastric volume, or motility disorder
2. NCLEX® Points
   a. Assessment
      i. heartburn
         1. exacerbated by bending over, straining, or recumbent position
      ii. regurgitation
      iii. hypersalivation
      iv. difficulty swallowing
      v. dyspepsia (discomfort in upper abdomen)
   b. Therapeutic Management
      i. Diagnosis made via pH test, esophagoscopy used to rule out malignancy
      ii. do not eat within 2 hours of bedtime

   iii. avoid food that reduce lower esophageal sphincter tone

    1. peppermint

    2. chocolate

    3. carbonated beverages

    4. smoking

    5. fried and fatty foods

   iv. eat a low fat, high fiber diet

   v. avoid medications that ↓ gastric emptying (anticholinergics)

   vi. elevate HOB while sleeping

   vii. Medications

    1. antiacids

    2. H2 receptor antagonists

    3. Proton pump inhibitors

Peptic Ulcer Disease

1. Overview

  a. Break in mucosal lining of stomach, pylorus, duodenum, or esophagus that come in contact with gastric secretions

2. NCLEX® Points

  a. Assessment

   i. pain

    1. Gastric

     a. gnawing, sharp 30-60 after a meal

    2. Duodenal

     a. 1.5 to 3 hours after eating

     b. relieved by eating

   ii. Upper GI series and EGD used to diagnose

   iii. hematemesis (gastric)

   iv. melena (duodenal)

  b. Therapeutic Management

   i. avoid foods that cause irritation

    1. coffee

    2. cola

    3. tea

    4. chocolate

    5. high sodium

    6. spicy foods

  ii. smoking cessation

  iii. small, frequent meals

  iv. avoid aspirin and NSAIDs

  v. monitor H&H and assess for bleeding

  vi. Surgical options

    1. gastrectomy

    2. vagotomy

    3. gastric resection

    4. Bilroth I, Bilroth II

  vii. medications

    1. H2 receptor antagonists

    2. Proton pump inhibitors

    3. Antacids

    4. sucralfate (Carafate)

Hiatal Hernia

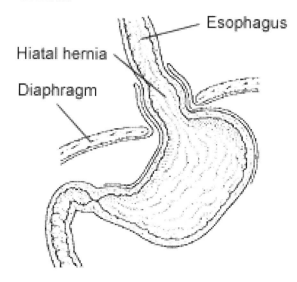

1. Overview

  a. Protrusion of bowel through the diaphragm into thorax

  b. due to weakening of muscles in diaphragm

2. NCLEX® Points
    a. Assessment
        i. heartburn
        ii. regurgitation
        iii. dysphagia
        iv. fullness
        v. bowel sounds over chest
    b. Therapeutic Management
        i. similar to GERD
        ii. do not lay down for 1 hour after eating
        iii. avoid medications that delay gastric emptying (anticholinergics)
        iv. eat small, frequent meals
        v. avoid straining
        vi. avoid vigorous exercise
        vii. sleep with HOB elevated

Inflammatory Bowel Disease (IBD)

Ulcerative Colitis

1. Overview
    a. chronic inflammation of mucosa and submucosa in colon and rectum
    b. results in poor absorption of nutrients
    c. progresses upward from rectum to cecum
    d. perforation may develop as colon becomes edematous leading to lesions and ulcers
    e. exacerbation and remission episodes
2. NCLEX® Points
    a. Assessment
        i. 10-20 liquid stools per day containing blood and mucus
        ii. malnutrition, dehydration, electrolyte imbalances
        iii. anorexia
    b. Therapeutic Management
        i. Maintain NPO during acute phase administering IV fluids and electrolytes
        ii. reduce intestinal activity
        iii. assess stool

        1.   assess for blood
- iv. monitor for bowel perforation and hemorrhage
- v. diet therapy
  1. low residue
  2. high protein
  3. high calorie
  4. vitamins and iron
- vi. avoid foods that may exacerbate symptoms
  1. raw vegetables and fruits
  2. nuts
  3. popcorn
  4. whole-grain
  5. cereals
  6. spicy
- vii. medications
  1. corticosteroids
  2. salicylates
  3. immunomodulators
  4. antidirrheals

Crohn's Disease

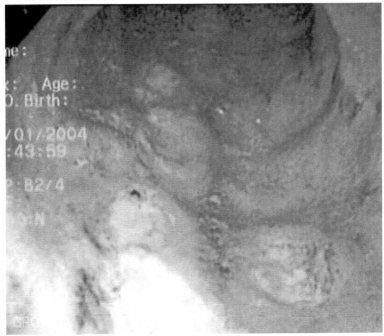

By Samir at English Wikipedia [GFDL (http://www.gnu.org/copyleft/fdl.html) or CC-BY-SA-3.0 (http://creativecommons.org/licenses/by-sa/3.0/)], via Wikimedia Commons

1. Overview
   a. inflammatory disease of GI mucosa anywhere from mouth to anus most often affecting the terminal ileum
   b. leads to thickening and scarring, ulcerations and abscesses
   c. remissions and exacerbations
2. NCLEX® Points
   a. Assessment
      i. fever
      ii. cramps and pain after meals (relieved by defecation)
      iii. diarrhea containing mucus or pus (5-6 stools/day)
      iv. anemia
      v. electrolyte imbalances

vi.   malnutrition
b.   Therapeutic Management
    i.   diet
       1.   high calorie
       2.   high protein
    ii.   medications - similar to ulcerative colitis
    iii.   weigh daily and maintain accurate I&O

Appendicitis

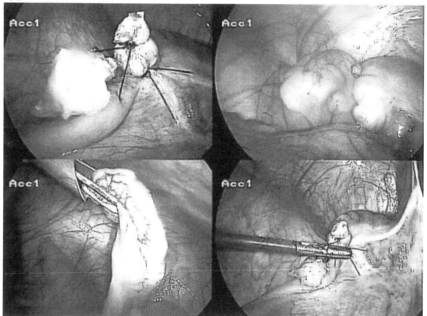

1.   Overview
    a.   Inflammation of the appendix
    b.   major risk factor is appendix rupture leading to peritonitis and/or sepsis
2.   NCLEX® Points
    a.   Assessment
       i.   abdominal pain at McBurney's point
       ii.   pain descends to RLQ
       iii.   ↑WBC
       iv.   rebound tenderness
       v.   fever

      vi.   abdominal guarding

     vii.   sudden relief of pain indicates rupture

  b.   Therapeutic Management

      i.   Appendectomy

        1.   keep client NPO

        2.   avoid heat application which can lead to rupture

        3.   avoid stimulation of peristalsis

        4.   if rupture occurs, postoperative healing is prolonged will have drains and NG tube for decompression

        5.   monitor VS and assess for abdominal distention post operatively

Diverticulitis and Diverticulosis

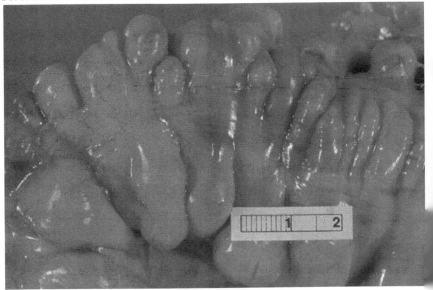

1.   Overview

  a.   Diverticulosis

      i.   Outpouching of intestinal mucosa

  b.   Diverticulitis

      i.   Inflammation of one or more diverticulosis due to trapped food or bacteria can lead to perforation and peritonitis

2. NCLEX® Points
    a. Assessment
        i. LLQ pain worsening with straining
        ii. ↑temp
        iii. N/V
        iv. Abdominal distention
        v. Melena
    b. Therapeutic Management
        i. NPO - bowel rest
        ii. bedrest
        iii. introduce fiber slowly
        iv. ↑ fluid intake
        v. avoid gas forming foods
        vi. bulk forming laxatives
        vii. avoid nuts, foods with small seeds

Hemorrhoids

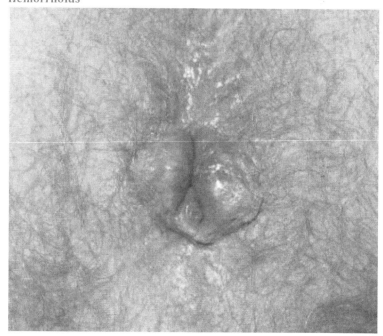

1. Overview
    a. swollen and inflamed veins of the anus and lower rectum

      b.   caused by straining, portal hypertension, irritation

      c.   internal, external, or prolapsed

2.   NCLEX® Points

      a.   Assessment

            i.   rectal pain

            ii.   bright red bleeding with defecation

      b.   Therapeutic Management

            i.   sitz-bath

            ii.   high fiber diet

           iii.   ↑ fluid intake

           iv.   stool softeners

            v.   cold packs and analgesics

Cholecystitis
1. Overview
   a. acute or chronic inflammation of the gall bladder most often caused by gall stones (cholelithiasis)
2. NCLEX® Points
   a. Assessment
      i. N/V
      ii. RUQ pain
         1. can occur 2-4 hours after high fat meals
         2. lasting 1-3 hours
      iii. Murphy's Sign
         1. pain with expiration while examiners hand is placed below the costal margin on right side at midclavicular line. Patient then asked to inspire if patient is unable to inspire due to pain, test is positive.
      iv. rebound tenderness
   b. Therapeutic Management
      i. NPO
      ii. antiemetics
      iii. nasogastric decompression
      iv. analgesics
      v. avoid gas forming foods
      vi. surgery
         1. cholecystectomy
            a. removal of gall bladder
            b. monitor for pain and infection at incision site
            c. abdominal splinting when coughing
            d. T-tube
               i. High Fowlers position
                  1. report drainage >500mL

Hepatitis
1. Overview
   a. inflammation of liver
   b. severity varies from mild cases with liver cell regeneration to severe cases with hepatic necrosis and cell death within weeks
   c. Forms
      i. Hepatitis A (HAV)
         1. health care workers at risk
         2. Transmission
            a. fecal-oral
            b. person-to-person
            c. poorly washed hands/utensils
            d. contagious
               i. most contagious 10-14 days prior to onset of symptoms
            e. self limiting
         3. Prevention
            a. strict hand washing best preventative measure
            b. Hepatitis A vaccine
      ii. Hepatitis B (HBV)
         1. health care workers at risk
         2. Transmission
            a. IV drugs
            b. blood or body fluids
            c. sexual contact
         3. Prevention
            a. hand washing
            b. blood screening
            c. Hepatitis B vaccine
            d. needle precautions
            e. safe sex practices
      iii. Hepatitis C (HCV)
         1. health care workers at risk
         2. Transmission
            a. IV drug users

             b. blood
        3. Prevention
             a. hand hygiene
             b. needle safety
             c. blood screening
    iv. Hepatitis D (HDV)
    v. Hepatitis E (HEV)

2. NCLEX® Points
    a. Assessment
        i. Preicteric Stage
            1. flulike symptoms
            2. pain
            3. low grade fever
        ii. Icteric Stage
            1. jaundice
            2. ↑bilirubin
            3. dark urine
            4. clay colored stool
        iii. Posticteric Stage
            1. recovery phase
            2. laboratory values return to normal
            3. pain relief
            4. increased energy
        iv. Laboratory values
            1. ↑ALT, AST, Ammonia, Billirubin

Cirrhosis

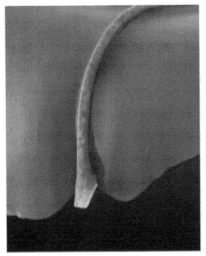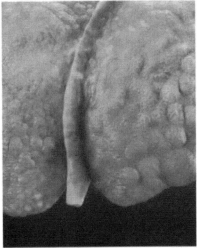

healthy   cirrhosis

1. Overview
    a. chronic, irreversible liver disease
    b. inflammation and fibrosis of liver cells (hepatocytes) leads to formation of scar tissue within liver which causes obstruction of hepatic blood flow and impedes proper liver function
        i. interruption of blood flow causes
            1. edema
            2. ascites
            3. esophageal varices
            4. hemorrhoids
            5. varicose veins

2. NCLEX® Points
   a. Assessment
      i. malaise
      ii. jaundice with scleral icterus
      iii. edema
      iv. anorexia
      v. clay-colored stool
      vi. pain in RUQ
      vii. hepatomegaly
      viii. splenomegaly
      ix. ascites (positive fluid wave test)
      x. hepatic encephalopathy
         1. disorientation
         2. altered LOC
         3. fatigue
      xi. asterixis (flapping hand tremor)
      xii. ↓reflexes
      xiii. anemia
      xiv. dark urine
   b. Complications
      i. portal hypertension
         1. increased pressure in portal vein
      ii. ascites
         1. fluid accumulation in abdominal cavity
      iii. esophageal varices
         1. dilated, thin veins in the esophagus can rupture
         2. bleeding is an life-threatening emergency
         3. goal is to control bleeding
      iv. Hepatorenal syndrome
         1. renal failure associated with liver failure
   c. Therapeutic Management
      i. elevate HOB
      ii. parecentesis to drain abdominal fluid
      iii. fluid restriction
      iv. ↓protein intake
      v. ↓ Na intake

          vi.   monitor daily weights

          vii. institute bleeding precautions and monitor coagulation studies

         viii. Medications

              1.   vitamin K

              2.   antacids

              3.   lactulose to decrease ammonia levels

              4.   analgesics

              5.   blood products

              6.   diuretics

Pancreatitis

1. Overview
   a. inflammation of the pancreas
   b. autodigestion of pancreas results
   c. Alcohol abuse, gall bladder disease, PUD, obstruction of the ducts and hyperlipidemia common causes
   d. Acute - occurs suddenly with most patients recovering fully
   e. Chronic - usually due to longstanding alcohol abuse with loss of pancreatic function
2. NCLEX® Points
   a. abdominal pain
      i. sudden onset
      ii. mid epigastric
      iii. LUQ
   b. N/V
   c. weight loss
   d. abdominal tenderness
   e. ↑WBC, bilirubin, ALP, amylase, lipase
   f. Cullen's sign
      i. bruising and edema around the umbilicus
   g. Turner's sign
      i. flank bruising
   h. steatorrhea
3. Therapeutic Management
   a. ↓pancreatic secretions
   b. NPO

      c.   NG tube insertion to decompress stomach and suppress pancreatic secretions

      d.   IV hydration

      e.   TPN for prolonged exacerbations

      f.   educate on avoidance of alcohol

      g.   notify provider of exacerbations

      h.   ERCP to remove gall stones

      i.   medications

            i.   analgesics

            ii.   H2 blockers

            iii.   Proton pump inhibitors

            iv.   insulin

            v.   anticholinergics

NCLEX® Cram - Gastrointestinal Disorders

1. Functions of the liver
   a. store vitamin B112 and fat-soluble vitamins
   b. store and release blood
   c. produce plasma proteins
   d. synthesize clotting factors
   e. convert amino acids to carbohydrates
   f. synthesize glucose
   g. detoxify alcohol and drugs
2. Functions of the pancreas
   a. secrete insulin and glucagon
   b. secrete sodium bicarbonate
   c. secrete pancreatic enzymes (amylase, lipase)
3. EGD
   a. keep client NPO for 6-12 hours prior
   b. keep client NPO until gag reflex returns
4. Colonoscopy

COLONOSCOPY

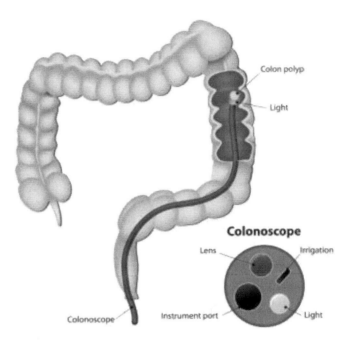

a.   position
    i.   side lying (left side) knees drawn up to chest
b.   colon must be clean prior to procedure

5. Paracentesis
    a. removal of fluid from the peritoneal cavity
        i. monitor vital signs closely
        ii. monitor breathing - rapid fluid removal can lead to shock
        iii. Position
            1. upright, back supported
        iv. measure fluid collected
6. Liver biopsy
    a. monitor for bleeding
        i. high risk for bleeding
    b. position post procedure
        i. right side
        ii. pillow under costal margin
7. GI Surgery
    a. Colonostomy
        i. low-residue (low fiber) diet
        ii. assess appearance of stoma
            1. notify provider if stoma becomes pale, darkened, cyanotic, or bleeding increases
        iii. insure proper fit of pouch
            1. 1/8 inch between stoma and bag
            2. empty bag when 1/3 full
8. Pernicious anemia
    a. body unable to absorb vitamin B12
    b. requires monthly B12 injections
9. Dumping syndrome
    a. complication of gastric surgery (common with Billroth I and II)
        i. rapid emptying of gastric contents into small intestine without proper digestion
        ii. symptoms begin 30 minutes after eating
        iii. N/V
        iv. abdominal fullness
        v. palpitations
        vi. tachycardia
10. BMI
    a. $BMI = wt\ (kg)/Ht^2(m)$

11. Malnutrition
    a. signs
        i. dry skin
        ii. anemia
        iii. muscle wasting
        iv. alopecia
        v. cheilosis (dry scaling lips)
        vi. glossitis
12. Melena - bloody stool
13. Steatorrhea - fat in stool
14. Intestinal obstruction
    a. assessment
        i. early - high pitched bowel sounds
        ii. late - absent
        iii. vomit with fecal scent
        iv. abdominal distention
    b. maintain NPO
15. Jaundice
    a. due to hyperbilirunemia
        i. bilirubin is a byproduct of hemoglobin breakdown
        ii. with liver damage bilirubin is not broken down
16. Ammonia
    a. byproduct of protein digestion in large intestine
    b. protein -> ammonia -> urea -> excreted via urine
    c. liver converts ammonia to urea
        i. with liver damage - ammonia levels raise in blood - causing complications and neurologic changes
        ii. lactulose draws ammonia from the blood into the urine to be excreted via stool
    d. BUN - measure renal and liver function
        i. ↑BUN = kidneys are not able to excrete urea
        ii. ↓BUN = liver is not converting ammonia to urea
17. Liver cancer
    a. RUQ pain, fatigue, anorexia, ascites, jaundice, liver failure
18. Pancreatic cancer
    a. causes
        i. smoking

    ii. toxins

    iii. high fat diet

  b. slow onset

  c. most clients do not present with symptoms until disease is advanced

  d. supportive care

  e. symptoms

    i. pain - worse when lying down

    ii. jaundice

    iii. weight loss

    iv. steatorrhea

19. Celiac Disease

  a. gluten sensitivity

  b. lifelong dietary modifications required

  c. Celiac Crisis

    i. acute episode

      1. precipitated by infection

      2. fasting

      3. gluten ingestion

      4. leads to: dehydration, electrolyte imbalance, severe acidosis

    ii. Assessment

      1. severe steatorrhea

      2. abdominal distention

      3. anemia

    iii. instruct patient on reading food labels

Metabolic and Endocrine Disorders

Syndrome of Inappropriate Antidiuretic Hormone (SIADH)

1. Overview
   a. Excess secretion of ADH from posterior pituitary leading to hyponatremia and water intoxication
   b. caused by trauma, tumors, infection, medications
2. NCLEX® Points
   a. Assessment
      i. fluid volume excess
         1. ↑BP
         2. crackles
         3. JVD
      ii. altered LOC
      iii. seizures
      iv. coma
      v. urine specific gravity >1.032
      vi. ↓BUN, hematocrit, Na+
   b. Therapeutic Management
      i. cardiac monitoring
      ii. frequent neurological examination
      iii. monitor I&O
      iv. fluid restriction
      v. Na supplement
      vi. daily weight (loss of 2.2 lbs or 1kg = about 1L)
      vii. Medication
         1. hypertonic saline
         2. diuretics
         3. electrolyte replacement

Diabetes Insipidus

1. Overview
   a. hyposecretion or failure to respond to ADH from posterior pituitary leading to excess water loss
   b. urine output ranging from 4L to 30L in a 24 hour period leads to dehydration
   c. Causes
      i. neurogenic, stroke, tumor, infection, pituitary surgery
2. NCLEX® Points

       a. Assessment
- i. excessive urine output
    1. dilute urine (USG <1.006)
- ii. hypotension leading to cardiovascular collapse
- iii. tachycardia
- iv. polydipsia (extreme thirst)
- v. hypernatremia
- vi. neurological changes

       b. Therapeutic Management
- i. water replacement
    1. D5W if IV replacement required
- ii. hormone replacement
    1. DDVAP (Desmopressin)
    2. Vasopressin
- iii. monitor urine output hourly and urine specific gravity
    1. report UO >200mL/hour
- iv. daily weight monitoring

Hyperthyroidism (Throtoxicosis)

1. Overview
   a. Excess secretion of thyroid hormone (TH) from thyroid gland resulting in **increased metabolic rate**
   b. Causes
   - i. **Graves disease** (autoimmune reaction)
   - ii. excess secretion of TSH, tumor, medication reaction
   c. Thyroid Storm (Thyroid Crisis)
   - i. extreme hyperthyroidism (life threatening) due to infection, stress, trauma
       1. febrile state, tachycardia, HTN, tremors, seizures
2. NCLEX® Points
   a. Assessment
   - i. ↑T3, T4, free T4, ↓TSH, positive radioactive uptake scan
   - ii. goiter
   - iii. bulging eyes
   - iv. Cardiac

       1. tachycardia, HTN, palpitations

   v. Neurological

       1. hyperactive reflexes, emotional instability, agitation, hand tremor

   vi. Sensory

       1. **exophthalmos** (Graves disease), blurred vision, heat intolerance

  vii. Integumentary

       1. fine thin hair

 viii. Reproductive

       1. amenorrhea, decreased libido

   ix. Metabolic

       1. increased metabolic rate, weight loss

3. Therapeutic Management
   a. provide rest in a cool quiet environment
   b. antithyroid medications (PTU, propylthiouracil)
   c. cardiac monitoring
   d. maintain patent airway
   e. provide eye protection
      i. regular eye exams
      ii. moisturize eyes
   f. Radioactive Iodine 131
      i. taken up by thyroid gland and destroys some thyroid cells over 6-8 weeks
         1. avoid with pregnancy
         2. monitor lab values for hypothyroidism
   g. Surgical removal
      i. monitor airway
         1. assess for obstruction, stridor, dysphagia
         2. have tracheotomy equipment available
      ii. maintain in semi-Fowlers position
      iii. assess surgical site for bleeding
      iv. monitor for hypocalcemia
         1. have calcium gluconate available
      v. minimal talking during immediate post operative period

Hypothyroidism
1. Overview
   a. hyposecretion of TH resulting in decreased metabolic rate
   b. Myxedema coma
      i. lifethreatening state of decreased thyroid production
      ii. coma result of acute illness, rapid cessation of medication, hypothermia
2. NCLEX® Points
   a. Assessment
      i. think HYPOmetabolic state
      ii. Cardiovascular
         1. bradycardia, anemia, hypotension
      iii. Gastrointestinal

        1. constipation
- iv. Neurological
  1. lethargy, fatigue, weakness, muscle aches, parethesias
- v. Integumentary
  1. **goiter, dry skin, loss of body hair**
- vi. Metabolic
  1. cold intolerance, anorexia, weight gain, edema, **hypoglycemia**

3. Therapeutic Management
    a. cardiac monitoring
    b. maintain open airway
    c. monitor medication therapy (overdose with thyroid
       medications possible)
    d. medication therapy
        i. levothyroxine (Synthroid)
    e. assess thyroid hormone levels
    f. IV fluids
    g. monitor and administer glucose as needed

Addison's Disease vs Cushing's Disease		
Body System	Addison's (Hypo)	Cushing's (Hyper)
Cardiovascular	Hypotension, tachycardia	Hypertension, signs of CHF
Metabolic	Weight loss	Moon face, buffalo hump
Integumentary	Hyperpigmentation (bronze)	Fragile, striae abdomen and thighs
Electrolytes	Hyperkalemia, hypercalcemia, hyponatremia, hypoglycemia	Hypokalemia, hypocalcemia, hypernatremia, hyperglycemia

Addison's Disease
1. Overview
    a. **hyposecretion** of adrenal cortex hormones
    b. decreased levels of glucocorticoids and mineralcorticoids
       leads to hyponatremia, hyperkalemia, hypoglycemia,
       decreased vascular volume, fatal if untreated
2. NCLEX® Points
    a. Assessment
        i. review chart above

        ii.   think HYPO secretion of adrenal hormones (steroids)
- b. Therapeutic Management
  - i. monitor vital signs
  - ii. monitor electrolytes (potassium, sodium, calcium)
  - iii. monitor glucose
    1. treat low blood sugar
  - iv. administer replacement adrenal hormones as needed
  - v. lifelong medication therapy needed
- c. Addisonian Crisis
  - i. caused by acute exacerbation of Addison's Disease
  - ii. causes severe electrolyte disturbances
  - iii. monitor electrolytes and cardiovascular status closely
  - iv. administer adrenal hormones as ordered

Cushing's Disease

1. Overview
   - a. **hypersecretion** of glucocorticoids leading to **elevated cortisol levels**
   - b. greater incidence in women
   - c. life threatening if untreated
2. NCLEX® Points
   - a. see chart above
   - b. ↑cortisol, Na+, glucose, ↓K+ and Ca++
3. Therapeutic Management
   - a. monitor electrolytes and cardiovascular status
   - b. provide skin care and meticulous wound care
   - c. provide for client safety
   - d. adrenalectomy (surgical removal of adrenal gland)
   - e. protect client from infection
   - f. often caused by tumor on adrenal gland or pituitary gland

Diabetes Mellitus

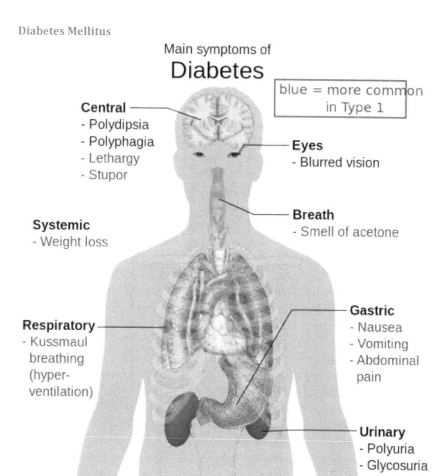

Main symptoms of

Diabetes

blue = more common in Type 1

Central
- Polydipsia
- Polyphagia
- Lethargy
- Stupor

Eyes
- Blurred vision

Breath
- Smell of acetone

Systemic
- Weight loss

Respiratory
- Kussmaul breathing (hyper-ventilation)

Gastric
- Nausea
- Vomiting
- Abdominal pain

Urinary
- Polyuria
- Glycosuria

1. Overview
    a. pancreatic disorder resulting in insufficient or lack of insulin production leading to elevated blood sugar
        i. **Type I (insulin dependent/juvenile-onset):** immune disorder, body attacks insulin producing beta cells with resulting **Ketosis** (result of ketones in blood due to gluconeogenesis from fat)
        ii. **Type II (insulin resistant/adult-onset):** beta cells do not produce enough insulin or body becomes resistant

2. NCLEX® Points
    a. Assessment
        i. 3 P's
            1. polyuria, polydipsia, polyphagia
        ii. elevate BS
        iii. blurred vision
        iv. elevated HgbA1C
        v. non healing wounds
        vi. neuropathy
        vii. inadequate circulation
        viii. End organ damage is a major concern due to damage to vessels
            1. coronary artery disease
                a. HTN, cerebrovascular disease
            2. retinopathy
    b. Therapeutic Management
        i. Insulin
            1. required for type I and for type II when diet and exercise do not control BS
            2. assess for and teach the patient regarding peak action time for various insulins
                a. only administer short acting insulins IV
            3. **study onset times and peak times for insulins**
            4. do not use expired insulin
            5. do not use a vial that appears cloudy (NPH exception)
            6. Mixing regular and NPH
                a. clear (regular) before cloudy (NPH)
                b. inject air needed into NPH, remove needle, inject air needed into regular, remove regular, remove NPH
        ii. patient should monitor BS before, during, and after exercise

      iii.   patient should use protective footwear to prevent injury

      iv.   infections and wounds should receive meticulous care

      v.   foot care

         1.   feet should be kept dry

         2.   footwear should always be worn

         3.   should not wear tight fitting socks

      vi.   sick day

         1.   continue to check blood sugars and **do not** withhold insulin

         2.   monitor for ketones in urine

      vii.   15 rule

         1.   if BS are low administer 15 gram CHO (5 lifesavers, 6 oz juice) recheck BS in 15 min

      viii.   Complications

         1.   lipoatrophy

            a.   loss of subq fat at injection site (alternate injection sites)

         2.   lipohypertrophy

            a.   fatty mass at injection site

         3.   Dawn phenomenon

            a.   reduced insulin sensitivity between 5-8am

            b.   evening administration may help

         4.   Somogyi phenomenon

            a.   night time hypoglycemia results in rebound hyperglycemia in the morning hours

Hyperglycemic Hyperosmolar Nonketotic Syndrome (HHNS)

1.   Overview

    a.   severe hyperglycemia without ketosis or acidosis

    b.   most often with type II

      c.   HHNS does not require the breakdown of fats for energy preventing ketosis. With HHNS enough insulin is available to breakdown carbs for energy.

2. NCLEX® Points

    a.   Assessment

        i.   gradual onset

            1.   infection, stress, dehydration

        ii.   altered LOC, dry mucous membranes

        iii.   BS >600 mg/dL

        iv.   negative ketones

        v.   ↑ BUN and creatinine

    b.   Therapeutic Management

        i.   determine cause

        ii.   replace fluids - may resolve hyperglycemia

        iii.   insulin therapy

        iv.   monitor neurological status

        v.   treat electrolyte imbalances

Diabetic Ketoacidosis (DKA)

1. Overview

    a.   severe insulin deficiency associated with type I diabetes

    b.   leads to the breakdown of fats into glucose resulting in ketones

2. NCLEX® Points

    a.   Assessment

        i.   sudden onset

            1.   infection, stress

        ii.   fruity breath

        iii.   ketones in urine

        iv.   hyperglycemia

        v.   dehydration

        vi.   acidosis (pH <7.35)

            1.   fats are broken down into glucose, ketones are by product of fat breakdown , ketones are acidic, potassium leaves the cell in attempt to compensate for acidemia

            2.   http://www.eric.vcu.edu/home/resources/consults/Hyperkalemia.pdf

       vii.   Kussmaul's respirations

      viii.   hyperkalemia

       ix.   ↑BUN and creatinine

       x.   monitor for altered LOC - cerebral edema can occur with fluid shift

  b.   Therapeutic Management

       i.   treat dehydration - with hyperglycemia water moves out of cells

       ii.   intensive insulin therapy

      iii.   monitor potassium

      iv.   assess for and treat acidosis

           1.   helpful to assess anion gap vs pH alone as pH takes into account respiratory effects view more here: http://www.merckmanuals.com/professional/endocrine-and-metabolic-disorders/diabetes-mellitus-and-disorders-of-carbohydrate-metabolism/diabetic-ketoacidosis-dka

NCLEX® Cram - Metabolic and Endocrine Disorders

1. Endocrine system
   a. hypothalamus
   b. pituitary gland (anterior/posterior)
   c. pineal gland
   d. thyroid gland
   e. parathyroid gland
   f. adrenal glands
   g. pancreas
   h. gonads
2. Endocrine system cheat sheet

Hormone	Gland	Under Production Syndrome	Over Production Syndrome
GH	anterior pituitary		acromegaly
ADH	posterior pituitary	diabetes insipidus	SIADH
T3,T4	thyroid	myxedema coma	graves
PTH	parathyroid	hyperparathyroid	hypoparathyroid
Glucocorticoids:	adrenal	addisons	cushings

cortisol			
Insulin	pancreas	diabetes mellitus	

3. Pituitary Gland Hormones
   a. ACTH
   b. FSH
   c. GH
   d. LH
   e. Prolactin
   f. TSH
   g. Oxytocin
   h. ADH
4. Radioactive Iodine Test
   a. measures thyroid function by measuring how much iodine is absorbed
      i. ↑iodine = hyperthyroidism
5. Glucocorticoids
   a. Cortisol
   b. blunt effect of insulin, suppress inflammation and immune response
6. Thyroid scan should not be completed on pregnant clients
7. Glucose Tolerance Test
   a. high level of glucose ingested
   b. glucose checked 2 hours after
   c. level >200 mg/dL suggests DM
8. HgbA1c
   a. indicates average plasma glucose concentration over time
   b. goal for diabetic clients is <7%
9. Transspehnoidal Hypophysectomy
   a. removal of pituitary tumor
   b. primary post operative concern is monitoring for nasal drainage
   c. assess for CSF in drainage using Halo Test
      i. blood in center with clear ring surrounding blood
   d. client **should not use a straw**
10. Pheochromocytoma
    a. tumor of the adrenal medulla
    b. causes excessive secretion of adrenal medulla hormones (epinephrine and norepinephrine)

      c.   HTN, palpitations, hyperglycemia, weight loss

      d.   avoid stimulation and provide constant cardiac monitoring

      e.   may need adrenalectomy

11. Parathyroid Disorders

      a.   think calcium

      b.   Hypoparathyroid = hypocalcemia

          i.   Trousseau's and Chvostek's signs

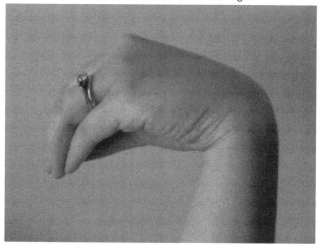

          ii.   provide calcium supplementation

          iii.   provide vitamin D which aids in calcium absorption

      c.   Hyperparathyroid = hypercalcemia

          i.   monitor for bone deformities

          ii.   renal calculi

Musculoskeletal Disorders

Osteoporosis

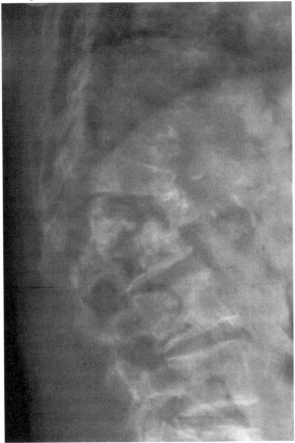

Clients with osteoporosis experience frequent fractures

1. Overview
   a. bone demineralization leading to ↓ bone mass
   b. bone resorption occurs faster than formation leading to Ca loss and porous bones
   c. more common in women due to ↓ estrogen
   d. high risk for factures
2. NCLEX® Points
   a. Assessment

        i. steroid use

       ii. female

      iii. ↓Ca intake

      iv. Kyphosis of spine

       v. bone pain

      vi. fractures of pelvis or hip

b. Therapeutic Management

       i. Ca+ intake and supplementation

      ii. Vitamin D intake

      iii. Weight bearing exercise

      iv. provide for a hazard free environment

       v. assistive devices

      vi. Medications

           1. alendronate (Fosamax)

           2. risendronate (Actonel)

           3. 30 minutes prior to eating

Osteoarthritis (Degenerative Joint Disease)

1. Overview

   a. progressive disorder of articulating joins

   b. affects weight-bearing joints and joints that receive a lot of stress (hands)

   c. Risk factors

       i. age, joint use, genetics

2. NCLEX® Points

   a. Assessment

       i. joint pain relieved with rest

      ii. Heberden's nodes and Bouchard's nodes

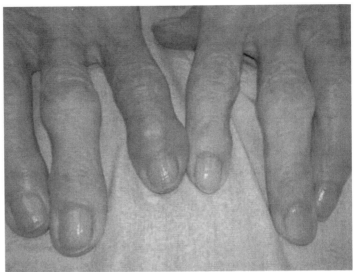

By Drahreg01 (Own work) [GFDL (http://www.gnu.org/copyleft/fdl.html) or CC-BY-SA-3.0
(http://creativecommons.org/licenses/by-sa/3.0/)], via Wikimedia Commons

   iii. difficulty standing up after sitting

   iv. crepitus in joints (grating sensation)

  b. Therapeutic Management

   i. administer pain medications

    1. topical agents

    2. NSAIDs

    3. muscle relaxants

   ii. corticosteroid injections

   iii. heat/cold applications

   iv. schedule rest periods

Gout

 1. Overview

  a. urate crystals deposit in joints and body tissues

  b. Hyperuricemia caused by ↑ purine synthesis, dietary intake, heredity, ↓ renal excretion of uric acid, alcohol intake

 2. NCLEX® Points

  a. Assessment

   i. painful joint inflammation and swelling

   ii. **Tophi**: nodules in skin

   iii. pruritus

        iv.   renal calculi
- b.   Therapeutic Management
    - **i.   Avoid purines**
        1. organ meat
        2. wine
        3. aged cheese
    - ii.   adequate fluid intake
    - iii.   bed rest during exacerbations
    - iv.   Medications
        1. anti-inflammatories
        2. antihyperuricemic: allopurinal (Zyloprim)

Rheumatoid Arthritis

1. Overview
    a. **Chronic** and **systemic** inflammatory disorder leading to weakened joints, dislocation, and deformity
2. NCLEX® Points
    a. Assessment
        - i.   inflammation of joints
        - ii.   joint stiffness
        - iii.   spongy joints
        - iv.   ↑ESR
        - v.   + rheumatoid factor
        - vi.   joint deformities
        - vii.   anemia
3. Therapeutic Management
    a. range-of-motion activities
    b. scheduled rest times
    c. heat/cold therapy
    d. paraffin baths
    e. assess clients reaction to body changes
    f. joint replacement possible (arthroplasty)
    g. medications
        - i.   NSAIDs
        - ii.   DMARDs
            1. Disease Modifying Antirheumatic Drug
                a. slow progression of disease
        - iii.   glucocorticoids

NCLEX® Cram - Musculoskeletal Disorders

1. Arthroscopy post procedure care
    a. assess neurovascular function
2. Bone resorption increases with age
3. Monitor site post biopsy for swelling, hematoma or pain
4. Strain - excessive stretching of muscle
5. Sprain - excessive stretching of ligament
    a. RICE
        i. Rest
        ii. Ice
        iii. Compression
        iv. Elevation

6.   Types of fractures

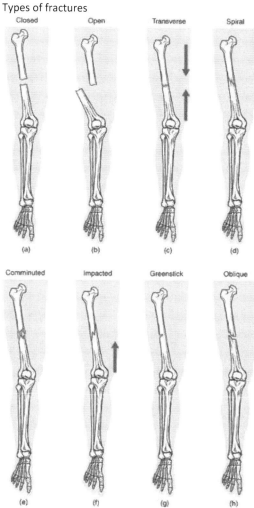

By OpenStax College [CC BY 3.0 (http://creativecommons.org/licenses/by/3.0)], via Wikimedia Commons

7.   Traction

    a.   force applied in opposite direction to immobilize fracture

    b.   insure the body is properly aligned

    c.   Buck's Traction

        i.   allow weights to hang from bed do not set them on floor

       d.   skeletal traction - uses pins inserted into bones
          i.   meticulous pin care required
       e.   Weights should not be moved by anyone

8. Casts
       a.   monitor extremity for swelling, pain, discoloration, loss of sensation, and pulse

9. Fat Embolism
       a.   risk with long bone fractures
       b.   originates in bone marrow and move into blood stream
       c.   patient may become tachycadiac and hypotensive
       d.   restless and tachypnea
       e.   emergent intervention is required

10. Compartment Syndrome
       a.   increased pressure within a body compartment usually with the arm or leg following trauma (fractures and crush injuries)
       b.   results in insufficient blood supply to the muscles and nerves
       c.   emergent surgery required to prevent loss of limb
       d.   Assessment
          i.   tissue becomes pale
          ii.   loss of sensation distal to injury
          iii.   pulseless
       e.   Fasciaotomy required to relieve pressure

11. Crutches
       a.   Going up Stairs
          i.   tripod position
          ii.   move unaffected leg up first
          iii.   move crutches and affected leg up next
       b.   Going down Stairs
          i.   move crutches down first
          ii.   move affected leg down next

12. Amputation
       a.   Phantom Pain
          i.   client has sensation of pain in amputated extremity
          ii.   can be treated with analgesics
          iii.   normal finding

13. Cane

       a.   Stand on affected side of client

       b.   hold cane on unaffected side

       c.   canes and crutches should have rubber stoppers on the bottom

14. Hip Replacement

       a.   proper body alignment must be observed postop

       b.   monitor for fat embolism

       c.   monitor wound and dressing for excessive drainage

15. Osteoporisis makes the client at risk for pathologic factures

16. Bone Scan

       a.   client should drink adequate fluids to flush dye from system

17. Vitamin D aids in Calcium absorption

18. Insure a safe environment for clients using walkers, canes, and crutches

Immunological Disorders

Anaphylaxis
1. Overview
   a. Severe allergic reaction with rapid onset with massive histamine release from damaged cells
   b. Life threatening if untreated
2. NCLEX® Points
   a. Assessment
      i. hives
      ii. angioedema (facial swelling)
      iii. respiratory complications
      iv. cardiac arrest
      v. hypotension
      vi. skin flushing
   b. Therapeutic Management
      i. assess client for allergies
      ii. assess respiratory and cardiovascular status
      iii. administer epinephrine
      iv. administer oxygen
      v. administer antihistamines
      vi. provide fluids as needed

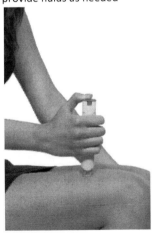

Systemic Lupus Erythematosus (SLE)

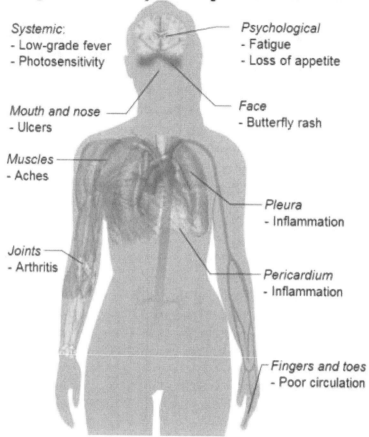

Most common symptoms of
Systemic lupus erythematosus

Systemic:
- Low-grade fever
- Photosensitivity

Psychological
- Fatigue
- Loss of appetite

Mouth and nose
- Ulcers

Face
- Butterfly rash

Muscles
- Aches

Pleura
- Inflammation

Joints
- Arthritis

Pericardium
- Inflammation

Fingers and toes
- Poor circulation

1. Overview
   a. progressive systemic inflammatory disease resulting in major organ system failure
   b. immune system "hyperactive" attacks healthy tissue
   c. no known cure
2. NCLEX® Points
   a. Assessment
      i. assess for precipitating factors

                        1. UV light
                        2. infection
                        3. stress
               ii. arthritis
               iii. weakness
               iv. photosensitivity
               v. Butterfly rash
               vi. ↑ESR and C Reactive Protein
       b. Therapeutic Management
               i. assess respiratory status
               ii. assess end organ function
               iii. plan rest periods
               iv. identify triggers
               v. refer to dietitian for dietary assistance
               vi. Medications
                        1. Glucocorticoids
                        2. NSAIDs
                        3. cyclophosamide (immunosupressive agent)

Acquired Immunodeficiency Syndrome (AIDS)

1. Overview
    a. Viral disease caused by HIV leading to spectrum of conditions
    b. Interferes with and destroys T4 cells making patient more susceptible to infections (TB, pneumonia, cancers, pneumonia)
2. NCLEX® Points
    a. Assessment
        i. Wasting syndrome
        ii. skin breakdown
        iii. frequent infections
        iv. stomatitis
        v. dehydration
        vi. malnutrition
        vii. leukopenia (↓WBCs)
        viii. Kaposi's sarcoma
               1. tumor caused by herpes virus
               2. purple/red lesions on skin and organs

    b.   Therapeutic Management
- i. respiratory support
- ii. nutritional support
  1. small frequent meals
  2. premedicate to avoid nausea
  3. provide favorite foods
- iii. monitor fluid and electrolyte balance
- iv. assess for infection
- v. provide skin care
- vi. initiate strict precautions and observe hand hygiene
- vii. conserve energy

Lyme Disease
1. Overview
   a. infection caused by tick bite
2. NCLEX® Points
   a. Assessment
      i. occur in three stages
      ii. flu-like symptoms
      iii. joint pain
      iv. neurological deficits
   b. Therapeutic Management
      i. remove tick
      ii. client should use bur spray prior to going outside
      iii. antibiotics must be taken as prescribed for the entire course
      iv. blood test can confirm diagnosis

NCLEX® Cram - Immunological Disorders
1. Innate Immunity
   a. present at birth
2. Acquired Immunity
   a. adaptive
      i. mother's antibodies
   b. active
      i. immunizations
3. Skin test
   a. discontinue taking antihistamines prior to test
4. assess all patient for latex allergy
5. clients with immunodeficiency are at a high risk for infection
6. patients who receive a transplant will have to take immunosuppressants for life
7. assess transplant patients closely for signs of rejection

Integumentary Disorders

Herpes Zoster (Shingles)
1. Overview
    a. viral infection seen in elderly individuals with a history of chicken pox
    b. occurs during immunocompromised state
    c. contagious to all individuals
2. NCLEX® Points
    a. vesicular rash
    b. fatigue, malaise, fever
3. Therapeutic Management
    a. isolation
    b. assess infection
    c. client may experience Bell's palsy
        i. assess neurological status
    d. Oatmeal bath may relieve itching
    e. Medications
        i. antivirals
        ii. NSAIDs
        iii. Shingles vaccination for elderly patients

Pressure Ulcers

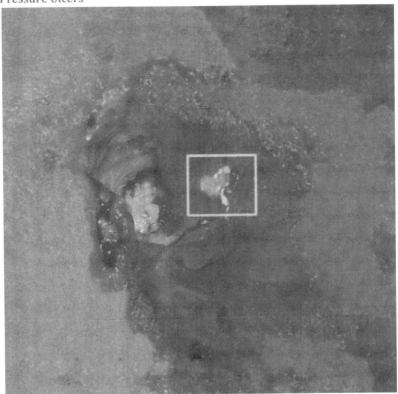

1. Overview
   a. excavations in the skin varying in size
   b. occur due to compression of tissue for extended period of time
2. NCLEX® Points
   a. Assessment
      i. Stage I
         1. skin is intact
         2. non blanchable redness
      ii. Stage II
         1. partial thickness loss of skin
      iii. Stage III
         1. full thickness skin loss extending to the dermis and subcutaneous tissue

          iv. Stage IV
1. full thickness skin loss exposing bone and muscle
2. undermining and tunneling
3. eschar may be present

       v. Deep Tissue Injury
1. subcutaneous tissue injury underneath skin

      vi. Unstageable
1. wound is covered by eschar or slough
2. unable to determine depth and thickness

b. Therapeutic Management
    i. **do not massage reddened area**
   ii. malnutrition, immobility, pressure are risk factors
  iii. assess patient skin integrity often
   iv. maintain skin dry
   v. turn patients q2h

Burns

1. NCLEX® Points
   a. Rule of 9s

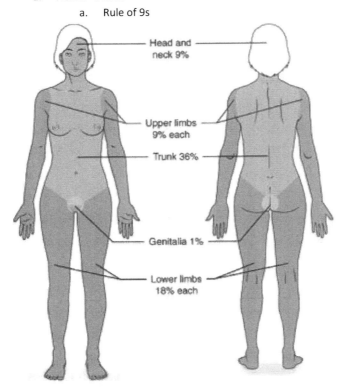

By OpenStax College [CC BY 3.0
(http://creativecommons.org/licenses/by/3.0)], via Wikimedia Commons

   b. Fluid resuscitation and infection prevention are the
      primary concern
   c. high calorie foods
   d. skin grafting
   e. monitor urine output - titrate fluid administration to urine
      output (30-50mL/hr)
   f. asses for edema

Skin Cancer

1. Overview
   a. abnormal cell growth

        b.   excessive exposure to sun
2. NCLEX® Points
        a.   Assessment
             i.   Asymmetry
             ii.   Border
             iii.   Color
             iv.   Diameter
             v.   Elevation
        b.   Therapeutic Management
             i.   Biopsy to confirm diagnosis
             ii.   instruct the client on risk factors
             iii.   educate on how to monitor lesions

NCLEX® Cram - Integumentary Disorders

1. Petechiae
        a.   small red spots that do not change color
2. keloid
        a.   irregular darker area of scar often seen with African Americans
3. MRSA (Methicillin-Resistant Staphylococcus Aureus)
        a.   contagious skin or wound infection that is spread by direct contact
        b.   maintain standard and contact precautions
4. Frostbite
        a.   rewarm with water and towels to salvage as much tissue as possible
5. Contact dermatitis
        a.   skin inflammation due to allergic reaction
        b.   Assessment
             i.   vesicles, bullae, erythema, oozing, scaling
        c.   Treatment
             i.   topical corticosteroids
             ii.   Burrow's solution
6. Stevens-Johnson Syndrome
        a.   drug induced skin reaction leading to the epidermis separating from the dermis
        b.   identify the cause, antibiotics, corticosteroids

Hematologic/Oncology Disorders

Anemia

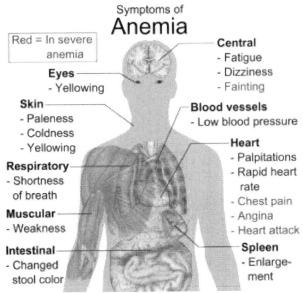

Symptoms of
Anemia

Red = In severe anemia

Eyes
- Yellowing

Skin
- Paleness
- Coldness
- Yellowing

Respiratory
- Shortness of breath

Muscular
- Weakness

Intestinal
- Changed stool color

Central
- Fatigue
- Dizziness
- Fainting

Blood vessels
- Low blood pressure

Heart
- Palpitations
- Rapid heart rate
- Chest pain
- Angina
- Heart attack

Spleen
- Enlargement

1. Overview
   a. ↓ in amount of RBCs or hemoglobin in blood, ↓ capacity of blood to carry oxygen
   b. Iron-Deficiency
      i. inadequate iron supply - 60% of anemias
   c. Pernicious
      i. Vitamin B12 deficiency
   d. Aplastic
      i. ↓ production of RBCs
2. NCLEX® Points
   a. Assessment
      i. pallor
      ii. weakness
      iii. cheilosis
      iv. spoonlike nails
      v. ↓MCV, MCH, Iron
      vi. Pica - craving clay and starch
      vii. Schillin test (for Pernicious anemia)

b.   Therapeutic Management
  i.   assess for occult blood
  ii.   monitory laboratory studies (Hgb, Hct)
  iii.   Increase iron intake in diet
      1.   green leafy vegetables
      2.   organ meat
  iv.   provide iron supplements
  v.   administer Iron via Z-track method
  vi.   take iron on an empty stomach
  vii.   limit visitors to patients with aplastic anemia

Sickle Cell Disease

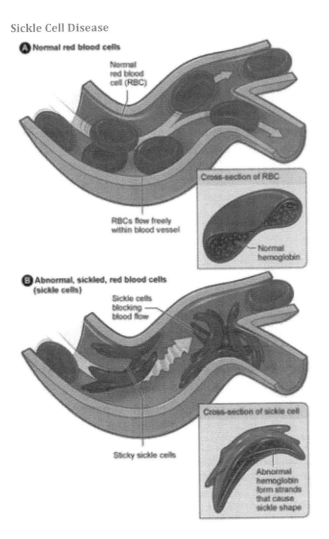

1. Overview
   a. hereditary disorder that affects the hemoglobin ability to carry oxygen leading to rigid, misshapen RBCs
   b. primarily affects African Americans by recessive trait
   c. can lead to sickle cell crisis due to hypoxia, exercise, high altitude, fever
2. NCLEX® Points
   a. Assessment

         i.   pallor

        ii. fatigue

      iii. severe pain

    b.   Therapeutic Management

         i.   supplemental oxygen

        ii. increase fluid intake

      iii. provide analgesia

      iv. blood transfusion

Thrombocytopenia

1. Overview

    a.   Decrease in circulating platelets (<100,000/mL)

    b.   Causes

         i.   decreased production

        ii. increased destruction

      iii. medication induced

2. NCLEX® Points

    a.   Assessment

         i.   ↓ platelet count

        ii. petechiae

      iii. bleeding (epistaxis, gi bleeding, melena, hematuria)

      iv. ↓Hgb, Hct

       v. monitor CBC

    b.   Therapeutic Management

         i.   platelet transfusions

        ii. Bleeding precautions

            1. avoid invasive procedures

            2. soft bristled toothbrush

            3. avoid medications that interfere with coagulation

            4. monitor for signs of bleeding

      iii. Diagnosis made via bone marrow aspiration

Disseminated Intravascular Coagulation (DIC)

1. Overview

    a.   widespread activation of the clotting cascade that results in the formation of blood clots in the small blood vessels throughout the body, normal clotting is disrupted and severe bleeding and hemorrhage occurs

2. NCLEX® Points
   a. Assessment
      i. pallor
      ii. ecchymosis
      iii. hematomas
      iv. hemoptysis
      v. melena
      vi. occult blood in stool
      vii. dyspnea
      viii. chest pain
      ix. hematuria
      x. anxiety
      xi. confusion
      xii. prolonged aPTT, PT, and thrombin time
      xiii. ↓platelets
   b. Therapeutic Management
      i. determine and treat underlying cause immediately
      ii. replace clotting factors
      iii. initiate bleeding precautions
      iv. monitor I&O

Leukemia

1. Overview
   a. proliferation of abnormal, undeveloped WBCs
   b. diagnosed by blood tests and bone marrow biopsy
   c. characterized by type of WBC affected
      i. Acute lymphocytic leukemia (ALL)
         1. 2-4 years of age
      ii. Chronic lymphocytic leukemia (CLL)
         1. 50-70 years of age
      iii. Acute myelogenous leukemia (AML)
         1. peak at 60 years of age
      iv. Chronic myelogenous leukemia (CML)
         1. incidence increases with age

2. NCLEX® Points
   a. Assessment

Common symptoms of
Leukemia

Systemic
- Weight loss
- Fever
- Frequent infections

Lungs
- Easy shortness
  of breath

Muscular
- Weakness

Bones or joints
- Pain or
  tenderness

Psychological
- Fatigue
- Loss of appetite

Lymph nodes
- Swelling

Spleen and/or liver
- Enlargement

Skin
- Night sweats
- Easy bleeding
  and bruising
- Purplish
  patches
  or spots

    i. weight loss
    ii. fever
    iii. infections
    iv. pain in joints
    v. fatigue
    vi. night sweets
    vii. easy bleeding and bruising
    viii. ↑WBC CLL and CML
    ix. ↓WBC ALL and AML
    x. Philadelphia chromosome in majority of CML
          clients
  b. Therapeutic Management
    i. chemotherapy and radiation
    ii. apply pressure to biopsy site
    iii. initiate neutropenic precautions
    iv. initiate bleeding precautions

      v.   reverse isolation
- 1. gown
- 2. glove
- 3. sterilize all equipment
- 4. strict hand washing
- 5. no fresh fruits or flowers

      vi. avoid fatigue
- 1. plan activities to provide time for rest

      vii. instruct client on oral hygiene
- 1. rinse mouth with saline
  - a. avoid lemon, alcohol base mouth wash

Lymphoma

1. Overview
   a. cancer or the lymphatic system
   b. classified by cell type many forms but Hodgkin's vs non-Hodgkin's (90% are non-Hodgkin's)
2. NCLEX® Points
   a. Assessment
      i. Reed-Sternberg cells - Hodgkins only
      ii. Positive biopsy
      iii. night sweets
      iv. fatigue
      v. enlarged liver, spleen, and lymph nodes
   b. Therapeutic Management
      i. Chemotherapy and/or radiation
      ii. assess for bleeding

NCLEX® Cram - Hematologic/Oncology Disorders

1. Warning signs of cancer
   a. CAUTION
      i. Change in bowel pattern
      ii. Unusual bleeding
      iii. Thickening of breast, testicle, skin
      iv. Indigestion
      v. Obvious change in mole
      vi. Nagging cough
2. Cancer Staging
   a. Stage 0: carcinoma in situ

        b.   Stage I: local tumor growth

        c.   Stage II: limited spreading

        d.   Stage III: regional spreading

        e.   Stage IV: metastasis

3.   Testicular Cancer

        a.   instruct client to perform monthly self examination

            i.   best preformed after warm shower

4.   Cervical Cancer

        a.   women should have regular gynecological examinations with Pap smear testing

5. Breast Cancer
   a. metastisis can easily occur via the lymph nodes
   b. diagnosis is made via biopsy or tumor removal
   c. Risk Factors
      i. early menarche or late menopause
   d. BSE (Breast Self Examination)
      i. perform monthly 7-10 days after menses
   e. Do not perform blood pressure checks or invasive procedures on an arm that has had a mastectomy
6. Prostate Cancer
   a. men after 50 should have regular prostate examinations
   b. removal of the prostate gland can be achieved via Transurethral Resection of the Prostate (TURP)
7. Hemophilia A and B are X linked recessive traits carried by females and demonstrated in males
   a. leads to prolonged clotting times
8. Neutropenia
   a. WBC <2000/mm3
      i. observe reverse isolation
      ii. observe strict hand hygiene
      iii. no fresh fruits, vegetables, or flowers

Eye, Ear, Nose and Throat Disorders

Strabismus

1. Overview
   a. eyes do not properly align with each other
   b. due to lack of ocular muscle coordination
2. NCLEX® Points
   a. Assessment
      i. cover-uncover test
      ii. squinting
   b. Therapeutic Management
      i. patch good eye 1-2 hours daily
      ii. surgical repair

Amblyopia

1. Overview
   a. also referred to as lazy eye involves decreased vision in an otherwise normal appearing eye
2. NCLEX® Points
   a. signs of visual impairment
   b. diagnosed by optometrist
3. Therapeutic Management
   a. corrective lenses
   b. cover good eye a few hours daily

Glaucoma

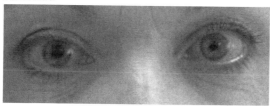

By James Heilman, MD (Own work) [CC BY-SA 3.0 (http://creativecommons.org/licenses/by-sa/3.0) or GFDL (http://www.gnu.org/copyleft/fdl.html)], via Wikimedia Commons

1. Overview
   a. Optic nerve damage caused by increased intra ocular pressure
   b. Two main categories
      i. Open-angle

      1. painless

      2. develops slowly

      3. no symptoms until advanced

   ii. Closed-angle (medical emergency)

      1. sudden eye pain

      2. redness

      3. vomiting

      4. sudden spike in intraocular pressure

2. NCLEX® Points

   a. Medication

      i. miotic drugs to constrict pupils

   b. requires lifelong drug therapy

   c. avoid medication that dilate pupils

      i. atropine

      ii. mydriatics

   d. institute safety measures for poor vision especially at night and in low light

Cataracts

1. Overview

   a. Clouding of the lens leading to decrease in vision

   b. risks include age, smoking, injury, DM

2. NCLEX® Points

   a. Assessment

      i. vision changes

      ii. loss of color vision

      iii. clouding of pupil

      iv. halos

      v. absence of red reflex

   b. Therapeutic Management

      i. surgery for removal of lens one eye at a time

      ii. patient safety is a priority

      iii. assist with ADLs

      iv. instruct client on eye protection

Detached Retina

1. Overview

   a. retina peels away from underlying support tissue

   b. medical emergency

2. NCLEX® Points
   a. Assessment
      i. sensation of curtain covering vision field
      ii. painless
      iii. gray retina
   b. Therapeutic Management
      i. the goal is to find and repair retinal breaks
      ii. lay client with affected side dependent
      iii. protect client from injury

Ménière's Disease
1. Overview
   a. disorder of the inner ear affecting hearing and balance
2. NCLEX® Points
   a. Assessment
      i. vertigo
      ii. tinnitus
      iii. hearing loss
      iv. head ache
   b. Therapeutic Management
      i. ↓Na intake
         1. ↑Na intake can exacerbate symptoms
      ii. bedrest
      iii. cochlear implant
      iv. endolymphatic sac decompression: create shunt for fluid drainage

NCLEX® Cram - Eye, Ear, Nose and Throat Disorders
1. Myopia
   a. nearsightedness
2. Hyporopia
   a. farsightedness
3. Closed Angle Glaucoma
   a. sudden eye pain with N/V
4. Never remove a penetrating object from the eye
5. Chemical splash
   a. flush the eyes for 15-20 minutes
6. Never use ear candles to remove cerumen
7. Rinne Test
   a. hearing test used to evaluate unilateral hearing loss

         b.   vibrating tuning fork on mastoid bone

8.   Weber Test

         a.   used to detect unilateral conductive hearing loss

         b.   vibrating tuning fork placed in middle of forehead

Your Free Gift!

As a way of saying thanks for your purchase, I'm offering a free PDF download:

"**63 Must Know NCLEX® Labs**"

With these charts you will be able to take the 63 most important labs with you anywhere you go!

You can download the 4 page PDF document by going to NRSNG.com/labs

Visit NRSNG.com to learn more and to get NCLEX® Cheat Sheets

29661790R00085

Made in the USA
Middletown, DE
26 February 2016